# Enjoy
# Life with
# Idiopathic
# Scoliosis during
# Adolescence

Psychology for
professionals of scoliosis

# Enjoy
# Life with
# Idiopathic
# Scoliosis during
# Adolescence

Psychology for
professionals of scoliosis

Elisabetta D'Agata

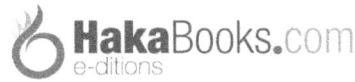

TITLE: *Enjoy Life with Idiopathic Scoliosis during Adolescence*
*Psychology for professionals of scoliosis*
AUTHOR: *Elisabetta D'Agata, 2019©*

LAYOUT: *HakaBooks - Optima, body 12*
COVER: *HakaBooks ©*

HAKABOOKS
*08204 Sabadell - Barcelona*
☎ *+34 680 457 788*
⌂ *www.hakabooks.com*
✉ *editor@hakabooks.com*
**f** *hakabooks*

Prohibited, within the limits established by law and under the warnings provided by law, the total or partial reproduction of this work by any means or procedure, whether electronic or mechanical, computer processing, rental or any form of transfer of the work without written authorization of the copyright holders.

All rights reserved.

*To adolescents with IS and their families.
And to my family and all my friends
who have supported me
on this adventure.*

"You are what people see when they arrive here.
Yours are the eyes they look into when they're frightened and lonely.
Yours are the voices people hear when they ride elevators, when they try to sleep and when they try to forget their problems.
You are what they hear on their way to appointments that could affect their destinies, and what they hear after they leave those appointments.
Yours are the comments people hear when you think they can't.
Yours is the intelligence and caring that people hope they'll find here.
If you're noisy, so is the hospital.
If you're rude, so is the hospital.
And if you're wonderful, so is the hospital.

(…)

We are judged by your performance.
We are the care you give.
The attention you pay.
The courtesies you extend.
Thank you for all you're doing".[1]

The president and CEO of Summa Health Systems in Ohio gave this statement printed in a wallet-sized card to all his employees reflecting values, beliefs and hope of the organization after interviewing all his workers.

---

1   Boyatzis R, McKee A. Resonant Leadership: Renewing Yourself and Connecting with Others Through Mindfulness, Hope and Compassion. Boston: Harvard Business Press; 2005

# CONTENTS

| | |
|---|---|
| Forewords | 13 |
| Acknowledgments | 17 |
| Introduction | 19 |

**FIRST PART - CENTERING ON PATIENTS**

| | |
|---|---|
| 1. FROM THEORY… | 27 |
| Integrating Models | 27 |
| Health Related Quality of Life | 30 |
| HRQOL in Adolescents with Scoliosis | 33 |
| The 10 Key Points of Chapter 1 | 39 |
| 2. TO PRACTICE: CONNECTING BEFORE CORRECTING | 41 |
| The Silence during the Medical Visit | 41 |
| The Body Doesn't Lie | 43 |
| The Mother | 49 |
| A Patient-Centered Communication | 52 |
| The Alliance | 57 |
| The 10 Key Points of Chapter 2 | 63 |
| The Decalogue for the First Visit | 65 |

**SECOND PART- ADOLESCENCE**

| | |
|---|---|
| 3. BODY | 69 |
| Body Image | 69 |
| The Embodiment Experience | 74 |
| Body Postures | 84 |
| Brace: The Challenge of a Crisis | 90 |
| Brace Wearing Preparation | 91 |

| | |
|---|---|
| Adherence | 94 |
| I Don't Want this Stuff!! | 98 |
| Traces of Brace | 99 |
| The 10 Key Points of Chapter 3 | 101 |
| **4. EMOTIONS** | **105** |
| Introduction | 105 |
| *I Don't Know* | 108 |
| Sadness | 114 |
| Shame | 117 |
| Fear | 122 |
| Anger | 126 |
| The 10 Key Points of Chapter 4 | 129 |
| **5. MIND** | **131** |
| The ESSENCE of Adolescence | 131 |
| Adults and Adolescents | 133 |
| Let Me Tell You a Story | 136 |
| A Hunchback God | 142 |
| Tales | 147 |
| Children to Adults: Rites of Passage | 151 |
| The 10 Key Points of Chapter 5 | 157 |
| **CONCLUSIONS** | **159** |

## *Foreword*

I had the privilege to meet Elisa years ago, when she came to Barcelona to write her Doctoral Thesis. I had the feeling, for a long time, that the quality of life of adults living their lives with a scoliosis was related, in some way, to the scoliosis they had but also to the way they 'wore' the scoliosis they had. At that time, I started to explain adolescent and their parents, when proposing any type of treatment strategy that most probably, for their future quality of life, it would not be so relevant the end result in terms of a particular angular value, but the way we, forming a team, were able to manage the whole situation, looking always for converting it into a positive experience. I always thought that creating nocebo expectations to adolescent, even with the best intention of looking for treatment compliance, was a bad strategy.

I am convinced that this book that Elisa has created, from her own personal experience, but finely structured in the best way from her long academic and professional background, will become a classic into the collection of books of all those professionals, doctors, physiotherapists, orthotists and psychologists, working in the field of Adolescent Idiopathic Scoliosis. She tells us about the importance of the Bio-Psycho-Social model, the importance of looking at the adolescent as a full person in the way of becoming a healthy, functional and mature adult. It is our responsibility to collaborate with the family in achieving this important objective. I advocate for young doctors, physiotherapists, Orthotists and Psychologists getting a humanistic education, and this precious book will help very much on this task. It is not just about psychology; it is about human rights.

Elisa, thank you very much for this contribution, which will help all of us to develop better in our profession.

*Manuel Rigo*
Medical Doctor, PhD
Rigo- Quera- Salvá Institut
Barcelona, Spain

Elisa has given us wonderful insight into the human side of AIS. In this book she gives us tools to observe the people who come to us for help with scoliosis, empathize with them and connect with them where they are. Using her suggestions which are backed by scientific research, we should be able to serve these individuals and help them achieve their potential, not only with the exercise program but in their wholeness as they mature and move from adolescence into adulthood. Her own personal experience with scoliosis and her years as a psychologist working with this population have given her a rich insight into the journey. These concrete tools will help professionals to assist adolescents while they navigate the challenges.

*Beth Janssen*
Physical Therapist
Certified BSPTS/SBI Instructor
Scoliosis Rehab Inc – President
Stevens Point, Wisconsin

Elisa has done a beautiful job of navigating the challenges of the head and the heart of the adolescent scoliosis patient. Her work goes beyond the structural and sterile stereotypes that unfortunately may come with AIS. She dives deeper into the person, not the patient.

I've been following Elisa's work for just a few years, but in that time, I've seen her passion shine through. Her understanding of the Bio-Psycho-Social (BPS) elements has helped not only her patients, but other professionals like me.

Every time I see Elisa present, I learn something new. Her compassion for people connects her academic and professional experiences seamlessly. This book is a resource for all of us. It's thoughtful, insightful and most of all, human. But then again this is Elisa, so I'm not surprised it's so hard to put down!

*MS, CPO (UK), CO (US), Grant Wood*
*Medical Doctor, PhD*
*Align Clinic, LLC*
*CEO and Co founder*
*San Mateo, California*

The following work, by the passionate author Elisabetta, invites us into a creative journey, without a doubt to redefine Scoliosis in teen years, through a scope of harmony and hope.

We can have a deep Bio-Psycho-Social (BPS) understanding in the treatment.

On her investigation, intervention and vision as a Psychologist and Psychotherapist, the author suggests an inclusive and Integrative model, where the teenager has a voice, and is co-author in the process of self-regulating and finally transforming.

This way Scoliosis becomes itself an internal dialogue, between oneself, its biography, emotions, self-perception, and the possibility of a new narrative.

This transformation goes way beyond an anatomical matter or about the cure of a pathology.

By abandoning the cartesian model, this proposal provides, dare I say, an antidote to this era of «Chronical Illnesses», thus making this way professionals more humanized instruments, with a more personalized approach to each case, creating safe bond states, constructing deep bridges between the psychological, neurological, biological, emotional, behavioral systems and their secondary benefices as an engine to the teenager patient.

Integrating the macro-vision since the beginning, where the contact with one self, the family system as well as their surroundings, will amplify the perception of the whole process.

A proposal that without a doubt will not leave indifferent the several professionals working on the treatment Idiopathic Scoliosis in teenagers, thus opening a window of opportunity of new abilities to a new field of intervention in this and other similar areas.

*Maria del Mar Cegarra Cervantes*
Clinical Psychology, M A,
Psychotherapist in Biosynthesis
Specialist in Psychosomatic, Epigenetics
and Neural Biology
Lisbon, Portugal

## *Acknowledgments*

I really would like to thank the following institutions and people:
The patients, for their full participation and for sharing their stories, emotions, questions and love, touching me deeply and teaching me a lot.
Vall d'Hebron Research Institut (VHIR) and Vall d'Hebron Hospital (Barcelona), especially the Traumathology Department, the Unit of Raquis, mainly Dr. Joan Bagó, for giving me the opportunity to experience the world of scoliosis from the hospital; Dr. Judith Sánchez-Raya from the Rehabilitation Department for all of her help and support; the physiotherapists, mainly Laura Franco, for their kind cooperation. All their voices still accompany me, inspiring me to think creatively.
Dr. Manuel Rigo, from Institut Rigo Quera Salva Institut, Barcelona, for his precious advice, giving me hope.
Dr. Carles Pérez-Testor, MD, Specialist in Psychiatry, Professor in Ramon Llull University, Barcelona for encouraging me to pursue this field.
All my family, María del Mar Cervantes, Rabieh Adib, Dr Ana Belén Vega, Beth Janssen, Grant Wood and all my friends and colleagues, for their enthusiastic encouragement and support.
Maria Caterina Miraglia, Angela Helmer, Beth Janssen, for their advice and revision.
All of you who are reading this book, for your interest. I look forward to hearing from many of you through my email: dagata.e@gmail.com

# *Introduction*

*We are souls in progress.*
*We were not born with a predestinated soul.*
*We are making our soul along the way.*
**–Enrique Vargas**

For the sensitive age of adolescence and the specificity of Idiopathic Scoliosis (IS) and its treatment, professionals of scoliosis may face several common problems related to communication, adherence to the treatment and the general stress of adolescent patients. So, as means of coping, these patients and the whole family system can present a variety of psychological issues such as worries, anxiety, disinterest, apathy, stress and more.

The goal of this book is to help those who work with adolescent patients with scoliosis, especially physical therapists who spend a lot of time with them, but also medical doctors, orthopedic technicians and psychologists, who are recently entering this field.

*Enjoy Life with Idiopathic Scoliosis during Adolescence* deals with the problems related to communication, motivation, emotions and adolescence, according to the bio-psycho-social framework, which integrates the biomedical model with the psychosocial one. As in the scoliosis field, there is not yet a concrete bridge from the theoretical framework to the professional practice, the application of the model remains unclear, up to individual and personal interpretation, without any clear guide, in a difficult attempt for the professional.

Starting from the vision that "every problem is an opportunity in disguise," as US President John Adams said, the idea behind this book is to transform our difficulties into powerful questions: How can we create favorable circumstances to offer the best treatment for our patients? How can we change passive adolescents into motivated ones? How can we respond to their emotional reactions? How can we establish a pleasant relationship? How can we get their parents to relax? This book offers some theories, intertwined with practical experience, in order to manage the difficulties in the treatment of our patients.

Professionally, in 2007 with my PhD course in Psychology, I started studying the Quality of Life of Adolescents with IS, in Barcelona and Milan, and then I worked in Vall d'Hebron Hospital in Barcelona for seven years. The hospital was a great opportunity to observe several medical visits of teenagers and adults with Idiopathic Scoliosis and also to work directly with them. I considered myself a privileged observer. It was as if a light was pointed on patients with scoliosis and I had the task to observe them, their familial relationships, their interactions with professionals, etc. Hundreds of patients were paraded in front of me and I literally took photos of most of them. As a psychologist and psychotherapist trained in Biosynthesis, for every patient, I could see their irregular waist, the curved column, but also those frightened eyes and above all I could hear a deep heavy silence. I asked myself how we could transform a medical visit, physical therapy or a brace treatment, from a standardized procedure into a rich, connected human process in favor of healthy growth of adolescents with scoliosis.

For this purpose, this book aims at enriching our scientific professionalism with kind and caring human communication to give us insight about how an adolescent may feel, think and behave. It is an integration between theory and lived experiences, offering clinical cases and work proposals for those who accompany these adolescents. I will be sharing some theoretical information, my professional experience and my personal involvement to help you in your work with adolescents with scoliosis.

First, regarding theories, I will present the bio-psycho-social model, the Health Related Quality Of Life concept and Patient Centered Communication (Chapter 1); for its application, timeless theories put forward by Palo Alto School are applied providing practical suggestions and the structure of the first session with the patient and his family (Chapter 2). Furthermore, recent science backed concepts related to body image are introduced (Chapter 3) as well as theories about emotions (Chapter 4) and adolescence brain development (Chapter 5) mostly originating from the advances of neuroscience. They can all enrich our knowledge and understanding of the experience of adolescents in scoliosis treatment and have an impact on our relationship with our patients during treatment.

Second, from my professional experience, I am pleased to share all my observations, notes and work proposals coming from my work with these patients. I would like to suggest an alternative manner of meeting patients, like the spotlight that lights up the radiographs and the surface topography exams may be complemented with our ability to accompany the family system, to create a bond and light up the patients, to understand their emotional world, to awaken their vital sparks in such a complicated situation. We have to go beyond the literal: raising our eyes from the examined radiograph, searching our patient's eyes, understanding implicit meaning in the family's communication, using humor, refining intuition, improving empathy. "Opening our mind like an umbrella"[2], overlapping the information of statistically significant scientific studies with the uniqueness of the person that is in front of us - integrating medicine as a science with medicine as an art is our CHALLENGE.

How can we create the conditions to see beyond appearances? Where should we look so that we don't fall into fantastical attributions or false impositions?

With this goal in mind, I will offer you resources from different disciplines such as psychology, neuroscience, narrative, poetry, myths, etc. In each chapter I mention clinical cases (in white windows) and offer practical work proposals (in grey windows marked by the symbol ♯). I hope it will be useful for your daily practice to motivate the patients to accept treatment and to connect with themselves.

Third, I feel a personal commitment with these patients. When I was 13, I tried on a swimsuit and I noticed something strange about my hips: they were lopsided. I did not tell my mother right away, as I thought it was not important. When I finally did tell her, I was immediately brought to the doctor who pronounced those famous words: idiopathic scoliosis of the adolescent. I had to wear a Milwaukee brace. I only associated that name, Milwaukee, to the place where a famous serial killer dismembered his victims and hid them at the turn of the last century. If I try to remember those years I encounter a certain difficulty, as if a layer of fog hides the memories.

---

2   Vega, A.B. Abriendo la mente como un paraguas. Ahora León [Internet]. 2018 Dec. [Cited 2019 Feb 19]. Available from: http://www.ahora-leon.com/abriendo-la-mente-paraguas

Colors were opaque. There was no sound. Time stopped. The kitchen clock became covered in dust. There was only one thing that woke me from my hazy existence. Once a week I went to the theater workshop at school. It was my only redemption from the monotony of my life. I felt my body, its vitality and energy; I could express my creative side and I was not ashamed of myself. When I was 18 years old, and my brace disappeared, I expanded my creative expression to dance, feeling my body in a whole new way.

My experience brought me along this journey; as a joke of life, my commitment has been written curiously, as my name *Elisa* magically appears in the acronym of the title of this book: **E**njoy Life with Idiopathic **S**coliosis during **A**dolescence.

*Enjoy your reading!*

# First Part

## Centering on Patients

# Chapter I
# From theory: the Bio-Psycho-Social Model

*Every art should become science*
*And every science should become art*
**—Heinrich von Schlegel**

## Integrating Models

Iain McGilchrist[3], a psychiatrist and neuroimaging researcher, studying the functioning of the brain, focused on a crucial aspect: its "bipartite nature" or, as he called it, our "divided brain"[4]. The two hemispheres see the world very differently, producing "two kinds of worlds" (McGilchrist, 2001). The right hemisphere experiences the world as a big picture, a net of interconnections; it understands relationships and body language, it creates art, intuition and imagination. The left hemisphere experiences the world as a map made by fragmented and isolated entities; it sees the details, not the relationships and it understands a person as made up of parts. The left hemisphere *is not a reliable guide to the nature of the*

---
3   McGilchrist, I. The master and his emissary: The divided brain and the making of the Western world. New Haven: Yale University Press; 2009.
4   McGilchrist I. Paying attention to the bipartite brain. Lancet. 2011 Mar 26;377(9771):1068-9.

*world, the brain or the body*. Its mechanistic vision is better for understanding machines, but its practical vision is easy to understand.

Each hemisphere sees a vital aspect of the experience, however, relying on one alone is a mistake. In fact, science does not come only from the left hemisphere, but it lies in open-mindedness, flexibility and empirical observation of experience. Its origin *needs* creativity, starting from the right hemisphere, while its procedures of assessment are realized by the left hemisphere. Furthermore, "medicine is not about bodies, brains, or minds, but about human beings, their lives and experiences. (...) But in order to understand human beings, we need to know something of what are still called the humanities. (...) Medical education needs urgently to be brought back to the humanities out of which it once arose. (...) Don't get me wrong: detailed scientific knowledge is hugely important. We rely on such minute information to inform the bigger picture. But it is a necessary, not sufficient, condition, of being a good physician. Without a way of understanding and interpreting it at a deeper level, more detailed knowledge will achieve precisely nothing, and will lead us ultimately to let our patients down" (McGilchrist, 2011).

Coming from the Enlightenment knowledge and following the Cartesian tradition (1596-1650), the biomedical (BM) model split the body into its structured and physiological parts, dividing the mind from the body, which subsequently determined the type of care a patient receives and the doctor-patient relationship[5]. It is likely the product of the left hemisphere's work.

In 1977, for the first time, the American psychiatrist George Engel introduced the Bio-Psycho-Social (BPS) model

---

5   Solano, L. Tra mente e corpo. Milano: Raffaello Cortina ed; 2001

in his article *The need for a New Medical Model: A challenge for Biomedicine*, published in Science[6]. Engel's proposal was theoretically based on the idea that in nature all the systems, from the smallest micro system to the largest macro one in the cosmos, are nested and inextricably interconnected through continuous feedback loops[7]. The integration of these systems is extremely important in terms of understanding the patient's bio-psycho-social story[8].

The introduction of the Bio-Psycho-Social (BPS) model represents a change in medicine and marks a transition from the biomedical (BM) model. The BPS model does not separate systems, but it integrates bio-physiological and psychological systems: it seems to be the integration of the work of the left and right hemispheres.

The BPS model gives a vision of life as a network of living and interconnected systems, as a result of the influence of the systemic model, the theory of relativity by Einstein, Cybernetics, new ecological theories and so on.

In his book[9], McGilChrist states that the right hemisphere is the master and the left an indispensable master's tool, his emissary. However, the clever emissary usurps the wise master and the results are tragic.

The big challenge is to integrate the left and right hemispheres, objective and subjective realities, biomedical and

---

6   Engel GL. The need for a new medical model: a challenge for biomedicine. Psychodyn Psychiatry. 2012 Sep;40(3):377-96.
7   Smith RC, Fortin AH, Dwamena F, Frankel RM. An evidence-based patient-centered method makes the biopsychosocial model scientific. Patient Educ Couns. 2013 Jun;91(3):265-70.
8   Farre A, Rapley T. The New Old (and Old New) Medical Model: Four Decades Navigating the Biomedical and Psychosocial Understandings of Health and Illness. Healthcare (Basel). 2017 Nov 18;5(4). pii: E88.
9   McGilchrist, I. The master and his emissary: The divided brain and the making of the Western world. New Haven: Yale University Press; 2009.

psycho-social models, measuring Cobb Angle as well as assessing the patient's emotions, thoughts, interpersonal relationships, communication rules, etc. For this reason, it is necessary to have an integrated team of health care professionals working under the same roof, all trained according to the biopsychosocial model, speaking one common language when evaluating and treating patients[10].

## Health Related Quality of Life

Thanks to technological and pharmaceutical advances, many of the diseases considered acute become chronic, with a consequential increase of non-fatal, but incurable diseases. Therefore, nowadays, we live in an "era of chronic illness"[11]. With the increase of life expectancy, mortality and morbidity do not cover the complexity of a person's life situation as it is expressed by the World Health Organization (WHO). WHO defined Health (1948) as a state of "complete" physical, mental and social well-being and not merely the absence of disease or infirmity"[12]. This definition overcame the negative concept of health as absence of disease and included the physical, mental and social areas of wellbeing.

The construct of Health Related Quality Of Life (HRQOL)

---

10 Wade DT, Halligan PW. The biopsychosocial model of illness: a model whose time has come. Clin Rehabil. 2017 Aug;31(8):995-1004.
11 Ambrosio L, Senosiain García JM, Riverol Fernández M, Anaut Bravo S, Díaz De Cerio Ayesa S, Ursúa Sesma ME, Caparrós N, Portillo MC. Living with chronic illness in adults: a concept analysis. J Clin Nurs. 2015 Sep;24(17-18):2357-67
12 Preamble to the Constitution of the World Health Organization as adopted by the International Health Conference, New York: World Health Organization, 19-22 June, 1946; signed on 22 July 1946 by the representatives of 61 States (Official Records of WHO, no. 2, p. 100) and entered into force on 7 April 1948.

is clearly an application of the BPS model. In fact, the World Health Organization defined the HRQOL[13] as a multidimensional construct (that embraces physical, mental and social domains), including the patient's perception, emphasizing its dimension of dynamic process over time (according to the age, the patient's life stage and the stage of the disease) and highlighting the importance of cultural factors in the process of self-evaluation.

Nowadays, the definition of "health" has been criticized, as the age of the population and the pattern of illnesses change. In 2011 Huber and colleagues[14] suggested a new meaning of health, as they considered the previous WHO's definition an unrealistic state of *complete* wellbeing in an ever aging world population with chronic diseases. "The requirement for complete health *would leave most of us unhealthy most of the time*". Furthermore, this group focused the attention on the dynamic dimension of health, rather than on the condition of 'a state'. They defined health as the *"ability to adapt and self- manage when individuals face physical, mental or social challenges"* or the resilience or capacity to cope and maintain one's integrity, equilibrium and sense of wellbeing. In this definition, coping with disease could be learned and the attention moves from what causes disease to what causes health.

As a consequence of this shift of perspective regarding

---

[13] World Health Organization Quality of Life (WHOQOL) Group. 1995. *The World Health Organization Quality of Life Assessment (WHOQOL): position paper from the World Health Organization.* Social Science and Medicine 41(10):1403-1409

[14] Huber M, Knottnerus JA, Green L, van der Horst H, Jadad AR, Kromhout D, Leonard B, Lorig K, Loureiro MI, van der Meer JW, Schnabel P, Smith R, van Weel C, Smid H. How should we define health? BMJ. 2011 Jul 26;343:d4163.

health, Alejandro Jadad, Professor of Toronto University, imagines *a pandemic of health* in his article[15]. Thanks to digital technologies, it is possible "to connect the best minds, the best knowledge, and the best tools across traditional boundaries to create a pandemic of health, and to improve the capacity of humans to imagine, create, and promote new and better approaches to living, healing, working, and learning". This vision is perfectly adaptable to societies with competent health professionals as well as Society on Scoliosis Orthopaedic and Rehabilitation Treatment (SOSORT), in their efforts to improve the treatments of scoliosis. What competencies do we need to provide successful treatments in the future? What should be avoided?

New words as *fun, passion, excitement and happiness* have entered science articles. This transformation is similar to the one present in psychology. Seligman and Csikszentmihalyi wrote[16]:"The exclusive focus on pathology that has dominated so much of our discipline results in a model of the human being lacking the positive features that make life worth living. Hope, wisdom, creativity, future mindedness, courage, spirituality, responsibility, and perseverance are ignored or explained as transformations of more authentic negative impulses". New questions and new constructs related to Positive Psychology arise as the following: What enables happiness? What are the effects of autonomy and self-regulation? How can optimism and hope affect health? What constitutes wisdom? How can talent and creativity come to fruition?

Coming back to our theme, my reflection is about how we,

---

15   Jadad AR. Creating a pandemic of health: What is the role of digital technologies? J Public Health Policy. 2016 Nov;37(Suppl 2):260-268.
16   Seligman ME, Csikszentmihalyi M. Positive psychology. An introduction. Am Psychol. 2000 Jan;55(1):5-14.

as professionals, can improve the patients' ability to face all the challenges scoliosis brings to their life. The consequence of the multi-dimensionality of the definitions of concepts as such as health and HRQOL, supports the idea that the treatment of scoliosis has to be multidimensional. It means that a conservative or surgical treatment has to include psychological and social components to follow the BPS model, maintaining a *Cartesian mechanical-reductionist* perspective.

## HRQOL in Adolescents with Scoliosis

From all of the above concepts, it is clear that we need, at our disposal, a repertoire of self-reported measures, as well as other tools, to better understand our patients. There is no easy answer to the question: "What is the best set of outcomes to use with patients with scoliosis?"

With an increasing number of HRQOL instruments being developed in general, and specifically in the scoliosis field, it is becoming difficult for researchers and clinicians to select the most appropriate instruments. Most of the time, the validations of the HRQOL tool or review studies report only basic properties of the instruments, as domains and psychometric properties, but not which conceptual background is below[17]: though there is not a single criterion standard for the HRQOL. The domains to measure the HRQOL differ, including emotional, social, physical health and well-being; items commonly assess difficulties or the frequency of feelings or symptoms, in contrast to positive aspects of life as we consid-

---

17   Davis E, Waters E, Mackinnon A, Reddihough D, Graham HK, Mehmet-Radji O, Boyd R. Paediatric quality of life instruments: a review of the impact of the conceptual framework on outcomes. Dev Med Child Neurol. 2006 Apr;48(4):311-8.

er in the last subchapter. Furthermore, the objective indicators of HRQOL, as in scoliosis, the Cobb Angle, generally have a poor relationship with subjective indicators, including multiple personality factors such as resilience, coping style and attitudes which can interfere. "Few quality of life instruments exist that focus on the positive aspects of adolescence, incorporate adolescents' perspectives and language, and apply to both general and vulnerable populations." [18] There appears to be a need to evaluate adolescents differently from adults. According to Frisén[19], the domains to assess adolescents are physical maturation and body image, peer relationships, intimacy and sexuality and autonomy.

Nowadays, in clinical research, the SRS-22 (Scoliosis Research Society)[20] is the most translated and widely used questionnaire to measure the HRQOL in both adults and adolescents. However, the SRS-22 is not a specific tool for adolescents as it lacks of specific adolescent issues. More specific tools, exploring the illness, as the ISYQOL (Italian Spine Youth Quality Of Life)[21] are being translated into several languages. Furthermore, graphic tests could be integrated with verbal ones, as in an increasingly visual society, adolescents catch images more easily than written texts[22]. The Trunk Appear-

---

18   Edwards TC, Huebner CE, Connell FA, Patrick DL. Adolescent quality of life, part I: conceptual and measurement model. J Adolesc. 2002 Jun;25(3):275-86.
19   Frisén A. Measuring health-related quality of life in adolescence. Acta Paediatr. 2007 Jul;96(7):963-8.
20   Asher M, Min Lai S, Burton D, Manna B. The reliability and concurrent validity of the scoliosis research society-22 patient questionnaire for idiopathic scoliosis. Spine. 2003;28(1):63-9.
21   Caronni A, Sciumè L, Donzelli S, Zaina F, Negrini S. ISYQOL: a Rasch-consistent questionnaire for measuring health-related quality of life in adolescents with spinal deformities. Spine. 2017;17(9):1364-1372
22   Matamalas A, Bagó J, D'Agata E, Pellisé F. Body image in idiopathic

ance Perception Scale (TAPS)[23] is a short tool which presents three sets of images exploring a trunk subjective perception.

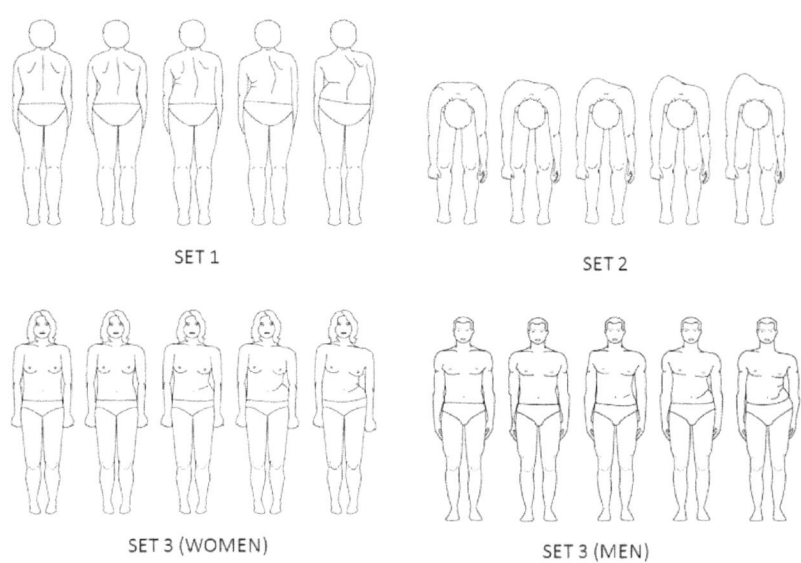

SET 1

SET 2

SET 3 (WOMEN)

SET 3 (MEN)

Despite the lack of time in our accelerated work life, clinicians could also use other instruments beyond the Patient Reported Outcomes (PRO) for assessing a patient's HRQOL. A psychosocial interview for adolescents such as **HEEADSSS**[24] treating specific issues of this period of life could be an inspiring means of exploration. This interview can be

scoliosis: a comparison study of psychometric properties between four patient-reported outcome instruments. Health Qual Life Outcomes. 2014 Jun 3;12:81

23    Bago J, Sanchez-Raya J, Perez-Grueso FJ, Climent JM. The Trunk Appearance Perception Scale (TAPS): a new tool to evaluate subjective impression of trunk deformity in patients with idiopathic scoliosis. Scoliosis. 2010 Mar 25;5:6.

24    Doukrou M, Segal TY. Fifteen-minute consultation: Communicating with young people-how to use HEEADSSS, a psychosocial interview for adolescents. Arch Dis Child Educ Pract Ed. 2018 Feb;103(1):15-19.

used in different ways and for different aims, for example: for an initial icebreaker to discuss hobbies and recent events; to deeply explore about risk-taking behaviors. If time is limited, it could be shortened and adapted. This interview should be directed to the adolescent alone, explaining to the parents that it is good for their child to start taking responsibility in their process of health treatment and creating a confidential and safe place for the adolescent to talk. A confidential discussion is required, with professionals assuring their patients of confidentiality to encourage an open and honest exchange by saying things such as "whatever you will say will be kept private between us, it will not be passed on to your parents or anybody else outside this office, unless you give permission" except that "If you tell me something that would put you at risk, I may have to speak to someone about it."

The interview is a guide to explore different areas of the patient's life and it can be used in a flexible way. The areas to explore are Home, Education/Employment, Eating, Activities, Drugs, Sexuality, Suicide/Low Mood, Safety (HEEADSSS). As a sample, you can see the following guide for the exploration of the Education area. See the five page article[25] to read the interview in its entirety.

---

[25] Doukrou M, Segal TY. Fifteen-minute consultation: Communicating with young people-how to use HEEADSSS, a psychosocial interview for adolescents. Arch Dis Child Educ Pract Ed. 2018 Feb;103(1):15-19.

HRQOL. A psychosocial interview for adolescents such as **HEEADSSS**[26] (#1#) treating specific issues of this period of life could be an inspiring means of exploration.

### #1#Fifteen-minute Consultation: HEEADSSS interview

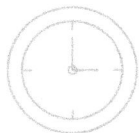

The interview is a guide to explore different areas of the patient's life and it can be used in a flexible way. The areas to explore are Home, Education/Employment, Eating, Activities, Drugs, Sexuality, Suicide/Low Mood, Safety (HEEADSSS).

It can be used in different ways and for different aims, for example: for an initial icebreaker to discuss hobbies and recent events; to deeply explore about risk-taking behaviors. If time is limited, it could be shortened and adapted. This interview should be directed to the adolescent alone, explaining to the parents that it is good for their child to start taking responsibility in their process of health treatment and creating a confidential and safe place for the adolescent to talk. A confidential discussion is required, with professionals assuring their patients of confidentiality to encourage an open and honest exchange by saying things such as "whatever you will say will be kept private between us, it will not be passed on to your parents or anybody else outside this office, unless you give permission" except that "If you tell me something that would put you at risk, I may have to speak to someone about it."

---

26  Doukrou M, Segal TY. Fifteen-minute consultation: Communicating with young people-how to use HEEADSSS, a psychosocial interview for adolescents. Arch Dis Child Educ Pract Ed. 2018 Feb;103(1):15-19.

As a sample, you can see the following guide for the exploration of the Education area.
Questions to ask your adolescent patient about Education:

» What school? What year?
» How do you feel in your school? Comfortable? Safe? Why?
» Have you ever been bullied?
» Do you have a best friend or a group of friends or prefer being alone?
» In your school are there any adults to trust?
» What is your best subject? Have you received any failing grades?
» How you see the future? what do you want to do?

See the five page article to read the interview in its entirety.

 In synthesis, the main points of this chapter are summarized below.

## The 10 Key Points of Chapter 1

1. The Bio-Medical (BM) model splits the body into its structured and physiological parts, dividing the mind from the body and considering disease as a deviation from the norm of measurable somatic variables.
2. The Bio-Psycho-Social (BPS) model is multi-causal and circular and also considers the human experience of a patient.
3. The biomedical model is not wrong but it is incomplete. The BPS model includes the biomedical model.
4. In 1948, "health" was defined (by WHO) as a state of "complete" physical, mental and social well-being and not merely the absence of disease or infirmity". This definition included the physical, mental and social areas of wellbeing.
5. In 1995, Health Related Quality Of Life (HRQOL) was described as a multidimensional construct that includes physical, mental and social domains.
6. In 2011, "health" was defined as the "ability to adapt and self-manage when individuals face physical, mental or social challenges" (**Huber and colleagues)**.
7. Recently, new concepts as *fun, passion, excitement, happiness, hope, wisdom, creativity, resources, etc.* enter science articles in medicine, as in psychology.

8. With an increasing number of HRQOL instruments being developed in general, and specifically in the scoliosis field, it is becoming difficult for researchers and clinicians to select the most appropriate instruments.
9. There is a need of evaluating adolescents differently from adult populations.
10. The assessment of an adolescent can be enriched by combining Patient Reported Outcomes (PROs) for Measurement of Health Related Quality Of Life with a specific psychosocial interview such as HEEADSSS. This instrument treats specific issues of adolescence as Home, Education/Employment; Eating; Activities; Drugs; Sexuality; Suicide/Low Mood; Safety (HEEADSSS).

# Chapter 2
## To practice: Connecting before correcting

> *If you talk to a man*
> *in a language he understands,*
> *that goes to his head.*
> *If you talk to him in his language,*
> *that goes to his heart.*
> **–Nelson Mandela**

### The Silence during the Medical Visit

When I worked in a hospital, I was present for medical visits for my work as a researcher. In a certain moment during the visit there was always a sacred silence devoted to the measurement of the last radiography. This silence weighed down on the parents' worries. Only the mother dared to break the silence with her legitimate question: "Doctor, has it (scoliosis) gotten worse?". The parents' questions expressed apprehension and worries: "How large is the curve? Doctor, will the curve increase?". On one side, the doctor attempted to measure the current radiographies, to compare them with the previous ones in order to evaluate the degrees of progression.

In some cases, the curve was larger, but the patient had

already reached the skeletal maturation and they probably would not grow any more. So the mother felt more relaxed and tried to ease the tension with a joke: " Doctor, so my daughter won't grow anymore!? She will stay a bit short then!". In this way, the attention passed from the radiography to the patient's height.

During this dialogue, the patients rarely intervened. They were measured, weighed, had to undress, etc. During this conversation between adults, the patients kept apart, seated abandoned on a chair, speechless, except when the doctor addressed them directly.

The doctor attempted to get the patient to speak, to create an atmosphere of silence in order to let the patient's shy voice be heard.

What a curious scene! It happened identically with many patients and their families. The same questions on the parents' side, the same lost gaze of the patient.

The adults' active roles, the patient's passive posture are meaningful non-verbal communication. I knew we could go deeper. Identifying the patients with their scoliosis is an act of reduction that cancels out any other question not specifically related to the spinal column. When everything has only one meaning, having only to do with the physical, there is nothing more to say. There are no explaining words, no tests, no questionnaires to measure what is happening in depth. I remained in silence while observing these interactions, with a sense of emptiness.

In these repeated scenes with different protagonists, it was very hard to reach the patient's emotional side. A barrier was expressed by a neutral response of "Well" or "I don't know," which separated the adolescent from the doctor, when he asked: *How are you?*

## The Body Doesn't Lie

A family enters our office, an outpatient clinic or a hospital for their first visit. It generally consists of a mother, father, the patient and sometimes other children or even a full matrilineal composition: grandmother, mother, daughter; or only a father and his daughter. They enter silently, respectfully, waiting to be received. The first moments of contact with another person are unique. First impressions can mark the dynamic of the entire relationship, as it happens in any relationship between two people, whether it is a professional relationship, friendship, or a future couple.

For this reason, we have to pay attention to the first moment when we meet our patients, above all, the place and the time of the meeting. When we think about the **place** where we are waiting for them we should ask ourselves: What is the space like where we meet our patients? Is it a silent, pleasant and intimate room or is it a noisy area with people coming and going and interrupting? Is it overly hygienic, cold and impersonal? What does it smell like? We should also think about the quality of **time** we devote to them, and consequently, on our presence during their visit. Do we look at them with attention or are we too busy with our computer or phone? What are our intentions and interest towards them and their stories?

The psychologist Albert Mehrabian[27] studied the importance of body language and intonation. What we say represents only 7% of communication while the rest of the message comes from how we are expressing ourselves: body language, facial expressions, voice inflection and the tone of our voice constitutes 93% of communication.

During our first meeting, we get in touch reciprocally.

---

27   Mehrabian, A. Non verbal Communication. Chicago: Aldine-Atherton; 1972.

Consequently, we have to make sure that we are communicating properly. If we really want to help our patients and their families who have come to our office, it is important to create a warm and friendly environment, taking care of them as if they are our guests. We have to welcome them, open the door, invite them to sit down and look at them smiling with genuine care and empathy.

We have to keep the first two of five axioms of the human communication in mind, elaborated by psychologist Paul Watzlavick[28] from Palo Alto, California. The first axiom of the Theory of Communication states that it is impossible not to communicate. One cannot *not* communicate. Everybody is communicating all the time. Even silence is a form of communication. This axiom emphasizes the important role of non-verbal communication. The second axiom follows, stating that communication has two levels: the first is the content of the message while the second, the non-verbal level, is about the *relationship*. Our voice, our facial expression are communicating something about the relationship with our client. So, the way we speak to our client about scoliosis influences the information we give, how the information is received and the relationship we are creating.

Moreover, when we meet a family, we have an opportunity to understand the family system, meaning the system in which our patient lives.

Regarding communication, Table #1# can be used as a tool to write your notes about the first meeting with the family. How do they communicate? Do they respect each other when they are speaking? Is there a silent person or a spokes-

---

28   Watzlawick P, Bavelas JB, Jackson DD. Pragmatics of human communication: A study of interactional patterns, pathologies, and paradoxes. New York: Norton; 1967.

person in the family? Do we feel harmony or tension? Do they agree or disagree in relation to some topics?

It is interesting to observe the following: How do they enter the room? What is our first impression? In which order do they sit? For example, does the couple sit together or does the patient sit in the middle? Does the father sit far from the rest of the family, while the mother is closer to the patient and to the professional?

There is an interesting research from the observational studies in animals, primates and human beings. Carney and other colleagues[29] studied the "expansion posture", the posture of taking space, stretching out. Making oneself big is related to power, dominance, risk taking behaviors and pain tolerance. While, the opposite, "contraction", is when we take up a small amount space, we wrap ourselves up. Becoming smaller reflects our feeling of powerlessness[30].

Does the manner in which they sit (staying relaxed in the chair or sitting on the edge of it) mean they are calm or stressed? Do they have an expansive or contractive posture?

---

29   Carney DR, Cuddy AJ, Yap AJ. Power posing: brief nonverbal displays affect neuroendocrine levels and risk tolerance. Psychol Sci. 2010 Oct;21(10):1363-8.

30   Carney DR, Cuddy AJ, Yap AJ. Review and Summary of Research on the Embodied Effects of Expansive (vs. Contractive) Nonverbal Displays. Psychol Sci. 2015 May;26(5):657-63.

| #1# Family's verbal and non-verbal communication |  |
|---|---|
| **First impressions** | |
|  | |
| **In which order do they seat? Spatial distance in the family** | (father, mother, patient) |
|  | |
| **Manners of getting seated and their postures** | (relaxed, anxious, apathic, collapsed, expansive, contractive, ...) |
|  | |
| **Types of communication** | (respectful, dominant, submissive, harmonious, tense, agreement, disagreement, ...) |
|  | |
| **Roles in the communication** | (spokesperson, silent person, ...) |
|  | |
| **Rate the quality of the relationship with patient's family** | (friendly, difficult, diffident, trusty, etc.) |
|  | |

Regarding the adolescents (Table #2#), our attention focuses on their physical distance from us and the possible emotions they can be experiencing (do they express fear or are they comfortable?), on their clothing style, on the way they speak (what are the qualities of their voice?). There are some patients I cannot hear clearly because their voice is too weak. Regarding their eye contact (who do they look at when they speak?), there are some patients who look at their mother when talking to us. Does their body present any micro-movements such as a trembling leg, nail biting, etc. Are these signs of tension?

It is also interesting considering incongruence between verbal and non-verbal communication. When there is an incongruence between the verbal and non-verbal, the latter is considered the most honest form of communication. If you ask to your patient "How is it going?", they say "Fine", but their expression is sad, trust their expression![31]

---

31   Morioka S, Osumi M, Shiotani M, Nobusako S, Maeoka H, Okada Y, Hiyamizu M, Matsuo A. Incongruence between Verbal and Non-Verbal Information Enhances the Late Positive Potential. PLoS One. 2016 Oct 13;11(10):e0164633.

| #2# Adolescent's verbal and no verbal communication ||
|---|---|
| **Posture and its related emotions** | (shyness, fear, comfortable, powerful, etc.) |
| | |
| **Appearance and clothing** | (teenage style/childish, fashionable, tidy, shabby, etc.) |
| | |
| **Bodily micromovements** | (nail biting, trembling legs, eye tremors, etc.) |
| | |
| **Voice** | (strong, feeble, dominant, depressive, happy, tense, tremulous, etc.) |
| | |
| **Quality of sight** | (sad, curious, vital, interested, elusive, etc.) |
| | |
| **Congruence or incongruence** | (between verbal and non-verbal communication) |
| | |
| **Rate the quality of the relationship with your client** | (friendly, difficult, diffident, trusty, etc.) |
| | |

## The Mother

The roles of mothers and fathers can be expressed very differently in families, however, I am describing my own personal experiences with some patients and their families and I have tried to capture the family dynamics that I often observed while treating patients.

In my experience, the mother usually sits on the edge of a chair and she is not at all quiet. The patient and the father sit more comfortably. The mother is the spokesperson of the family, charged with the task of communicating with the outside world: she is the mediator between the inside and outside of the family system. She is the most stressed because she reflects the worries of the whole family. Furthermore, she has to face a professional she does not know and who she has probably looked for herself. In this way she takes on the trans-generational role of the caretaker of the children. This is why she is stressed; she needs someone able to support her, but her husband might not be able to, either because he is absent or because her anguish is so overwhelming that he needs to protect himself from all that negativity. Sometimes the mother is desperate because she has already experienced the same story personally and she still remembers the torture of her painful back; she would be ready to wear the brace herself in place of her child because that Milwaukee brace or the Harrington rod horribly frightened her during her youth: these visits are a reminder making her relive the trauma that marked her adolescence.

These mothers often come to the office very frightened for their child. Fear makes them speak without pause, like a stream overflowing after a storm, or on the contrary, they stay silent, waiting to hear what the professional has to say. In the face of fear, we can act by creating a security zone for the family by asking questions and listening to them either in the case of a mother overflowing with words or in complete silence. Listening to her fears, letting her get all of her ghosts out: her most horrific nightmares about monstrous deformation, the difficulty of childbearing in the future if her daughter is the patient, the possible risks of surgery such as paralysis, ending up in a wheelchair, etc. After all of that, we can reassure them with our attention. It is really important that the mothers can express their fears and feel that they are being listened to. Only when the flowing of fear is under control and the state of anxiety has decreased because they have been listened to, we can start explaining and sharing our knowledge about scoliosis in a simple, comprehensible way.

We cannot ignore the silent father and adolescent either, as they have become spectators of the mother's anxiety. They are not stronger than her; they only embody different roles of the same family script they are playing. They observe the scene and they may appear detached. There are also fathers (or mothers) who are not interested and they are silently watching the show of their wives (or husbands), or ex-wives (or ex-husbands). We have to try to include them in our conversation, so that they can feel a part of the group; at the same time the fearful wives (or husbands) can feel like they are not alone and have someone who they can share their anguish with.

Only then we can start our visit, our exploration and our questions about our patient's clinical history. Table #3# is a suggestion to create a first contact with our adolescent patients.

| #3# Questions for your patient to create a first contact with him ||
|---|---|
| **Life domains of adolescent patient** ||
| School | Favorite subjects; relationship with schoolmates; teachers; etc. |
|  |  |
| Hobby | Extracurricular activities |
|  |  |
| Sport | Type, weekly frequency, competitions, etc. |
|  |  |
| Playing musical instruments | Type of instruments, private versus group classes; etc. |
|  |  |
| Favorite music | Which one? Listening every day? Going to concerts? etc. |
|  |  |
| Reading | Kind of favorite literature; last book read; favorite books; etc. |
|  |  |
| Drawing | Drawing media / techniques, drawing subjects, etc. |
|  |  |
| Volunteering | Type, frequency, etc. |
|  |  |

## A patient-centered communication

Usually in the beginning, the family gives a lot of information about the medical history. The parents describe the signs they observed before consulting us and any cases of scoliosis in the family history, etc., trying to give as much information as possible. The shy patients usually give short, appropriate answers often in monosyllables. Maybe they are astonished by the inexplicable diagnosis because it is idiopathic, because the attention of their families is suddenly directed to them, even if they do not feel any pain. As we use a patient-centered communication and not a disease-centered model, our attention is focused on both the family and the patient. Here is an easy decalogue for communication.

**Point 1: The patient is our 'target' while the parents are our allies.** The first step of our communication is turning our attention to the parents, but also including the patient with eye contact and language.

Believing that because the patients are children, they do not understand us, or because we do not have enough time to explain everything to them and we can let their parents explain to them later, is a big mistake and prevents us from establishing a good relationship with the patient.

On the other hand, we want to know who our patients are and although they have the same scoliosis as other patients, to us they are unique, made up of *more than the sum of their Cobb degrees*. For this reason, before talking about scoliosis, it is important to direct our attention toward their life, asking questions about their life domains: daily life, interests, favorite music, hobbies, school, friends, classmates and social life. In this case, Table ♯3♯ or the HEEADSSS interview (chapter 1) can be a useful tool, especially for exploring Education or Activities.

**Point 2: Using metaphors.** When speaking about scoliosis, we have to use a language that is easily understandable for people of every age, social class and cultural background. For this reason, using **metaphors** may be an effective form of communication because metaphors help to bring the unknown to the familiar[32]. If we explain scoliosis by talking about a twisted tree and representing the brace as a stick to support this tree, there is a good chance of being understood by everyone. In your office you can keep old braces to show to your new patients, as many have never seen a scoliosis brace before.

**Point 3: Normalizing and De-Pathologizing Scoliosis.** Using the right words, we have a good chance of reducing or even preventing parents' possible anxiety in relation to scoliosis.

We can normalize scoliosis by explaining that it is very common in nature among both animals and human beings. There are many famous people who have reached their goals despite their scoliosis, such as Usain Bolt, the fastest man in the world, or the violinist Yo-Yo Ma who underwent a scoliosis surgery, as well as models like Lourdes Ciccone, the daughter of the famous musician, Madonna.

Normalizing has an immediate effect on anxiety. In my workshops, when I introduced myself to the teenagers attending classes, I usually informed them that I have scoliosis: they looked at me with surprise as if an adult with scoliosis could not be in good health.

I have an adult patient with difficult body image issues due to her scoliosis. She has problems accepting the harsh, insensitive questions of the horrified doctor who had to eval-

---

32  Hanne M. Diagnosis and Metaphor. Perspect Biol Med. 2015 Winter;58(1):35-52.

uate her for possible disability: "Madam, have you seen your scoliosis?! How can you breath?!". In an instant this doctor cancelled out all the progress we had slowly been making together about the acceptance of her body. It is a clear example of the nocebo effect of the language, "when words are painful."[33]

**Point 4: Use simple and clear language.** For fruitful communication, especially during the first visit, the best is not to use technical words. In the beginning, words such as Risser or Cobb are not meaningful to patients. Some people talk about percentage instead of angles: "My daughter has 35% scoliosis". Technical words interfere in the doctor-patient relationship, which is so important for adherence to the treatment[34].

**Point 5: Promote Positive Body Image from the Beginning.** The word "deformity" comes from Latin *de-form*, that means "the alteration of form". It is generally used in scientific language as a neutral term for light, moderate or severe scoliosis. However, it could be considered offensive by patients who associate deformed people to monstrosities. I have personally heard it many times and I still hear this word being used. I have to confess that, in the past, I myself used this term, forgetting the patient does not know the scientific language: "Can you see your deformity?" Until one day I was astonished when a patient who reads my blog, commented on a post where I had used that word. She wrote: "Nobody will ever love us for that, for the deformity... It is only the word "deformity" that is cruel and inhuman... I had never contemplated

---

33   Benedetti F, Lanotte M, Lopiano L, Colloca L. When words are painful: unraveling the mechanisms of the nocebo effect. Neuroscience. 2007 Jun 29;147(2):260-71.
34   Kreps GL. Promoting patient comprehension of relevant health information. Isr J Health Policy Res. 2018 Sep 18;7(1):56.

using that word until few years ago on a control visit, when the doctor said to me: "You're always going to be deformed." It was hard that day for me".

Language can have a destructive charge and can cause real psychological damage to people. These words can be like arrows for a patient and can invite the person in front of the mirror to identify their asymmetry as a deformity. Without realizing it, the professional can function as a distorting mirror, impacting how the patients view themselves and the severity of their scoliosis. Alternatives terms to "deformity" can be used such as curve, deviation, alteration and asymmetry which are more neutral terms.

**Point 6: Give Patient Written Information.** The first visit is usually full of tension and families need to be informed. Unfortunately, the degree of online communication in the scoliosis field is not of high-quality.[35, 36] If we select materials to give to patients or write something to inform them about scoliosis, patients will rely on our written information to read at home as support.

**Point 7: Use Visual and Synthetic Information.** As we live in a highly visual culture, we can use different media to improve our communication with patients. I have seen graphics used to successfully explain the progression of Risser with age, graphics to explain the efficacy of the brace in relation with the

---

35   Nason GJ, Baker JF, Byrne DP, Noel J, Moore D, Kiely PJ. Scoliosis-specific information on the internet: has the "information highway" led to better information provision? Spine (Phila Pa 1976). 2012 Oct 1;37(21):E1364-9.
36   Wellburn S, Bettany-Saltikov J, van Schaik P. An evaluation of web sites recommended by UK NHS consultants to patients with adolescent idiopathic scoliosis at the first point of diagnosis. Spine. 2013 Aug 15;38(18):1590-4.

number of hours of treatment or spine models to explain the curve and its movements.

**Point 8: Tune In to the Adolescent's World.** We can use digital media such as Anatomy Apps, which are free online anatomical atlases to explain how our spine is made, to arouse curiosity and better inform patients.

Additionally, we can find YouTubers with scoliosis and Instagram accounts that explain scoliosis and encourage them to face it in the best possible way. The online website Scoliosus, "a web-based platform intended to empower scoliosis patients with the tools and resources they need to be successful brace-wearers"[37], is a great example.

Technology and social media are a huge part of the adolescents' worlds today. You only have to take care in choosing positive YouTubers or Facebook groups that show resilient faces and generously share good resources and support, as there are some who only share complaints, difficulties, anger and sadness.

**Point 9: Enter Softly into the Delicate World of Puberty.** With the development of the sexual body, shame is a very common emotion in adolescents. We have to be gentle when discussing delicate topics, especially if the professional is of the opposite gender to the patient. For example, a question about menarche should not be asked at the immediate beginning of the visit. Although, I know it is essential to understand the state of maturation and the risk of scoliosis progression, the girl would not understand its importance or relevance to her scoliosis and be put off by this sudden invasion of her privacy.

---

37   Scoliosis-us. Bracing for scolios-us [Internet]. [Cited 2019 Jan]. Available from: https://bracingforscoliosus.org

**Point 10: Asking for Permission for Physical Exploration.** It is important to explore the body of the patients after creating gentile contact with them and only after asking for permission. They could feel extremely vulnerable. It is helpful to creating a safe environment and assure their privacy. For example, some young boys or girls may be upset or embarrassed by the presence of a parent for the exam. Some young girls who do not yet wear a bra, but their bodies are developing, may feel obligated to withstand these seemingly infinite minutes frozen almost naked in front of a parent. I am sure some of them would like to collapse, escape or disappear in that moment. Our patients would greatly appreciate questions such as "Can I examine your back now? Is it ok for you? Do you prefer that your parents leave the room for the examination or do you want them to stay?".

## The Alliance

Although it seems that explaining all the information about scoliosis and its treatment is one of the most important aims of the first visit, if we do not create a trusting relationship with our client, it will be difficult for them to follow the treatment. Giving them all the information is important but it should be done after creating a good therapeutic alliance.

The therapeutic alliance should be the primary aim of the first visit. It is how we create a trusting relationship with our patients. The therapeutic alliance is related to the emotional bonds with our patient. In creating the alliance, we have to consider the needs and the concerns of the family, for example, giving them space to express and containing the mother's anguish, as discussed previously. The relationship itself is a third entity to be cared for, to be seen and heard. Furthermore, it has been asserted that the relationship is a central component in the adherence to treatment in different studies[38]. If you do not have a connection with a patient, it is common that they will have problems in adhering to the treatment. So, remember: **CONNECTING BEFORE CORRECTING!** Otherwise our efforts to help the patient might be in vain and they may not adhere to the treatment, which would be a waste of our professional competence. The treatment would most likely be very difficult. Again, the therapeutic alliance is an invitation to use our non-verbal communication (smile, warmth, eye contact, etc.) to make a real human connection with our patients and consequently make a real difference in their lives. Creating the alliance is a complex process that includes showing empathy, the exploration of expectations and the final agreement about goals and strategies[39] with our patients, which I will briefly describe below.

### a. Empathy or Putting Ourselves in Other People's Shoes

The neurons of empathy were first discovered in the early 1990s, when a team of Italian researchers found individual neurons in the brains of macaque monkeys[40]. Also called *mirror neurons*, they are a type of brain cells that respond equally when we perform an action and when we witness

---

38   Lambers NM, Bolton JE. Perceptions of the quality of the therapeutic alliance in chiropractic care in The Netherlands: a cross-sectional survey. Chiropr Man Therap. 2016 Jun 8;24:18.

39   Babatunde F, MacDermid J, MacIntyre N. Characteristics of therapeutic alliance in musculoskeletal physiotherapy and occupational therapy practice: a scoping review of the literature. BMC Health Serv Res. 2017 May 30;17(1):375

40   Rizzolatti G, Fadiga L, Gallese V, Fogassi L. Premotor cortex and the recognition of motor actions. Brain Res Cogn Brain Res. 1996 Mar;3(2):131-41.

someone else performing the same action. They have been localized in the frontal lobes of the brain, among motor command neurons, which is what they were originally thought to be. This research shows that empathy is an available resource present in everyone's brain.

Furthermore, the psychiatrist Siegel[41], Professor of Psychiatry at UCLA, defined empathy as the ability to create the mind-sight of another person, that means empathy is the ability to create a map of the mental life of another person. So when we are interested in what is happening in the mental life of our patients, we can wonder about their images, feelings, thoughts and sensations: in this way, we are tuning into their inner life and can better understand their behavior.

Additionally, there is an association between listening and empathy. In fact, empathic listening is one of the strategies of the art of communication[42]. Stephen Covey in his bestseller *7 Habits of Highly Effective People* wrote about the difficulty of empathic listening: "We are naturally inclined to want the opposite: we want to be understood first. Many do not even listen with the intent to understand; they listen with the intent to reply. They either speak, or they are ready to speak. Our conversations become collective monologues. We never really understand what is happening inside another human being."[43]

*Empathic behavior* diminishes anxiety, as a group of Swiss researchers demonstrated[44] by measuring the variation of cor-

---

41   Siegel D. Brainstorm: The Power and Purpose of the Teenage Brain. New York: Penguin Group; 2013
42   Buffington A, Wenner P, Brandenburg D, Berge J, Sherman M, Danner C. The Art of Listening. Minn Med. 2016 Sep-Oct;99(6):46-8.
43   Covey, S R. The 7 Habits of Highly Effective People: Restoring the Character Ethic. New York: Free Press, 2004.
44   Gemmiti M, Hamed S, Lauber-Biason A, Wildhaber J, Pharisa C,

tisol as stress response in medical interviews with 68 parents of pediatric consultations. When parents felt empathy from the professional, their cortisol levels decreased.

Scoliosis and its treatment are not easy for any patient to endure and adolescent patients are in a delicate period of development. Minimizing the effects on them of being diagnosed with scoliosis and going through the difficult treatments could be experienced by them as the professional being distant or insensitive, or it could separate the patient from their inner suffering. On the other hand, when we express understanding of their difficulties, we could help them to feel supported on their journey. It could be hard to listen to different patients with similar stories, but if we remain receptive to the patient (with empathic listening), we discover that they actually all have different and unique experiences, and this helps us to become more attuned and more fully understand their unique representation of their *mindsight*. Training ourselves in empathy is a useful exercise, not only at professional level, but also for our personal life, with our husband or wife, friends, children, parents, etc.

### b. Trust

Parents and patients trust us if they know that we are working in the best interest of the patient. Trust is also connected to confidentiality - the content of their visits is subject to professional confidentiality. There is no ambiguity about how this information can be used. When we speak with a patient we do not tell them about other patients unless we maintain their anonymity by not revealing personal details

---

Klumb PL. Pediatricians' affective communication behavior attenuates parents' stress response during the medical interview. Patient Educ Couns. 2017 Mar;100(3):480-486.

about the patient so they cannot be identified. This helps us to create a trusting relationship by maintaining confidentiality with all of our patients.

In regard to the relationship between the parents and the professional, frequently a parent reveals something about the private life of our patients while they are not in the room. They may reveal a "secret", for example that the patient is seeing a therapist or suffers from mental health issues, or is a victim of bullying, or is struggling with anorexia, etc. Knowledge of this secret puts us in a difficult position because it may be that the patients would not have revealed this to us themselves and feel that this is an intrusion of their privacy, thereby shutting down to open communication with the professional and putting the therapeutic alliance at risk. The best way out of this difficult situation is to first tell the parent that you will need to notify the patient of this knowledge and let the patient know that you have been informed of this personal information, without stating how you received this information, if possible, in order to maintain the alliance with both the parent and the patient. It is important to create an honest and open communication with our patient and the family. It is not healthy to keep a secret as that would be entering into, what may be, a very complicated family inner dynamics. Clearly state at the first visit that what the patient tells us remains between us, unless there is a serious risk for their life or other people's lives. This is an important ethical rule used to create a trusting relationship since the first visit.

### c. Agreement on Goals and Strategies

We have to work together with the parents, the patients, the doctors, the technical orthopedists, the psychologists - we are a collaborative team. In collaborative projects it is important to create an environment where people with different backgrounds, complementary skills, opposing personalities and work styles can all thrive.

In order to create an agreement with the patients and their families, it is important to explore their expectations, asking, for example: "How do you imagine our work together? Do you know people that go to physical therapy? How do you expect it to be?".

In this manner, they can express their expectations, whether realistic or unrealistic, and we can share our experience, explaining the treatment, negotiating responsibilities and giving them a more realistic vision of the treatment. For example, they could think that they do not have to do exercises at home, or that they have to use their brace only at night and they might be surprised by our presentation of the treatment plan, if we do it before discussing it with them.

After asking about their expectations, it is time to explain the session in detail, its duration, related homework and your fees. Then it is important to ask them if they agree with the how the sessions will be conducted and to make sure they understand what their responsibilities are outside of the sessions and agree to those terms as well. This creates a collaborative atmosphere where everybody is responsible.

After that we can discuss, in detail, the challenges of the treatment, for example the achievement goals, the amount of hours that they need to wear the brace or how much time they should dedicate to exercises and training, while remaining open to the possibility of negotiating, adapting the training to their schedule or their rhythm of life. It is important to ask: "Do you agree that we should consider a series of challenges to achieve? How do you want me to respond if you do not fulfill something that you have agreed to comply with?"

 In synthesis, the main points of this chapter are summarized below.

## The 10 Key Points of Chapter 2

1. First axiom of the Theory of Communication (Watzlavick). **It is impossible not to communicate.** Communication is a form of behavior. Everybody is communicating all the time. Even silence is a form of communication.
2. Second axiom of the Theory of Communication. **Communication has two levels.** The first is the content and the second is the non-verbal aspect. The non-verbal aspect represents the relational one.
3. **Our words constitute only 7% of the communication.** 93% of communication comes from body language and intonation (Mehrabian's study).
4. **Incongruence between verbal and non-verbal communication.** Non-verbal communication is the most honest form of communication. The *body doesn't lie*.
5. **The aims of the first visit are:**
   - To get to know the patient and their family (*Tables ♯1,2,3♯* are possibilities to record information from the first meeting)
   - To create an empathic relationship with the patient and the family, reducing anxiety
   - To explain what scoliosis is and its treatment in detail
   - To explore expectations about the treatment
   - To clearly state the rules of our work together
   - To check the commitment of our patient

6. **Connecting before correcting.** The Therapeutic Alliance is the emotional bond we create with our patients and their family. Starting a physical therapy without creating a human connection could be a problem for the patient's adherence to treatment. The ingredients of a therapeutic alliance are empathy, trust, checking their expectations and negotiating challenges.
7. **Empathy:** to create the *mind-sight* of our patients, that is, creating the map of their mental life to gain a deeper understanding.
8. **Trust:** working in the interest of the patient. It is also connected to confidentiality and to create a safe space where the patient can express themselves openly.
9. **Checking the patient's and parent's expectations about the treatment.** This gives us an idea of how far the patient wants to go into the therapy. *"How do you imagine our work together? Do you know people who go to physical therapy?"*.
10. **Negotiate challenges for treatment step by step.** This helps the motivation of our patients and enhances their commitment to achieve their objectives. For this last aim, ask questions such as: *"How do you want me to respond if you do not fulfill something that you had agreed to comply with beforehand?"*

An extra synthesis about the important role of communication on the first visit is reported below as a decalogue:

## The Decalogue for the First Visit:

1. **The patient is our 'target' while the parents are our allies.** In our communication with the parents we have always to include the patient as they are the center.
2. **Using metaphors.** Talking about scoliosis could be about an uncharted territory for patients and their families. Metaphors can be very useful, as they bring the unknown to the familiar.
3. **Normalize and de-pathologize Scoliosis.** The patient is not the only one with scoliosis. Scoliosis is present in nature. There are famous people with scoliosis who have achieved their dreams, as fashion models, athletes, actresses, musicians, etc.
4. **Use simple and clear language.** Avoid too much 'medical speak' during the first visit and explain any new terms beforehand. It could interfere with the patient's cognitive ability to understand the exchange, as well as with their relationship with you.
5. **Promote Positive Body Image from the beginning.** Use synonyms for "deformity", such as asymmetry, anomaly, alteration, deviation, curve, etc. In colloquial language "deformity" is a hard concept that can weaken the patient's body image.
6. **Give your patient written information.** The first visit is normally full of tension and sometimes the patient feels disoriented. Giving your patients written information to read at home is an act of care.

7. **Use visual and synthetic information.** Try to communicate and explain concepts appropriately for both the parents and the adolescent's cognitive development. Use concrete examples, such as graphics and avoid abstract concepts.
8. **Tune in to the adolescent world.** Use digital media such as Anatomy Apps, YouTubers, Instagram accounts, etc., to explain scoliosis and to encourage them to face it in the best way possible. Technology is a huge part of their world.
9. **Enter softly the delicate topic of puberty.** Ask about sexual development (Menarche and Turner's signs, etc.) directly to your patients, but only after having made good contact with them. Otherwise, patients might feel unnecessarily embarrassed and uncomfortable at the beginning of their first visit with their consultant.
10. **Explore the patient's body with care.** Examine the patient's body always asking for permission first. "Can I examine your back now? Is it ok for you? Would you prefer it if your parent isn't present during the examination?".

# Second Part

Adolescence

# Chapter 3
## Body

*The human body is the best work of art.*
—**Jess C. Scott**

*Take care of your body. It's the only place you have to live.*
—**Jim Rohn**

## Body Image

Body Image is an important issue for patients with Idiopathic Scoliosis and it has been assessed in several bodies of research, measured by different tools. Although it is considered especially important in the field of eating disorders (anorexia, binge eating disorder and bulimia), a commonly accepted definition of the concept is controversial while it has been considered as a multifaceted construct (Cash, 2004).

Body image is defined as a "multidimensional psychological experience of embodiment that comprises evaluative thoughts, beliefs, feelings and behaviors"[45]. Considering the multidimensionality of this concept, it is interesting to apply it to the world of scoliosis. The concept includes:

---

[45] Badoud D, Tsakiris M. From the body's viscera to the body's image: Is there a link between interoception and body image concerns? Neurosci Biobehav Rev. 2017 Jun;77:237-246.

**1. Perception of appearance** aspects: mental representation of size, shape and facial features. This point pertains to the "extent to which a person is able to judge his or her appearance accurately"[46].

Tools to assess the individual's degree of body size distortions have been developed, and in scoliosis, the Trunk Appearance Perception Scale (TAPS)[47] or the Spinal Appearance Questionnaire (SAQ) in its drawings[48] properly measuring the patient's perception;

**2. Attitudes** regarding body image encompass: A. Thoughts (beliefs about appearance, memories and assumptions); B. Feelings (emotions such as anger, happiness, sadness, etc.); C. Behaviors, such as camouflaging the body, clothing selection, changing body posture or body movements, avoiding looking at their own body, aesthetic treatments, etc.

A person with scoliosis, especially an adolescent, may struggle with a negative body image. Due to the fact that body image relates strictly to self-esteem and quality of life[49], professionals' concerns about a patient's body image can be explained.

---

46   Cash, T. F. Cognitive-behavioral perspectives on body image. In T. F. Cash & L. Smolak, editors. Body image: A handbook of science, practice, and prevention. New York: Guilford Press; 2011. p. 39-47.

47   Bago J, Sanchez-Raya J, Perez-Grueso FJ, Climent JM. The Trunk Appearance Perception Scale (TAPS): a new tool to evaluate subjective impression of trunk deformity in patients with idiopathic scoliosis. Scoliosis. 2010 Mar 25;5:6.

48   Sanders JO, Harrast JJ, Kuklo TR, Polly DW, Bridwell KH, Diab M, Dormans JP, Drummond DS, Emans JB, Johnston CE 2nd, Lenke LG, McCarthy RE, Newton PO, Richards BS, Sucato DJ; Spinal Deformity Study Group. The Spinal Appearance Questionnaire: results of reliability, validity, and responsiveness testing in
patients with idiopathic scoliosis. Spine. 2007 Nov 15;32(24):2719-22.

49   Sarwer DB, Polonsky HM. Body Image and Body Contouring Procedures. Aesthet Surg J. 2016 Oct;36(9):1039-47.

On the other hand, attitudes that patients have towards their own body affect the relationship between the Cobb degree and body image and a low-degree scoliosis can become a real problem for a patient while, on the contrary, a patient with severe scoliosis may not be negatively affected in regard to body image.

Furthermore, dissatisfaction to one's body image is a common psychological phenomenon assessed in Western society. The degree of dissatisfaction falls on a continuum from low to intense dissatisfaction that could be psychopathological, as in *body dysmorphic disorder* (BDD) (Sarwer & Polonsky, 2016).

It is necessary to consider the different levels of dissatisfaction with body image to identify possible problems with our patients. We may have patients who do not notice or care about their scoliosis when they look at themselves in a mirror. Although they have scoliosis, they have no problem with their body image. Because of their history, their background and the way they deal with emotions, they may live well, taking care of their spine with exercises, maintaining good posture, having positive feelings and thoughts toward their bodies. As well, there are those who do not like how their back looks, but they do not limit their activities and they come to accept themselves as they are. In the SRS-22 questionnaire, in item no. 19 it asks: "Do you feel attractive with your current back condition?", those patients may mark the answer: "Neither attractive nor unattractive". Their experience is neutral.

At the extreme end of this continuum, there are patients who look frequently at themselves in a mirror. They do not like what they see. They often look at themselves carefully and suffer from how they see themselves. Despite their friends or family trying to reassure them, they feel misunderstood and are greatly affected by their condition. So, they limit their activities by not going to the beach, not wearing tight clothing, not working out in the gym, not sitting in public with their back towards people, and so on. They often consider surgical treatments, if it is possible for them, but sometimes they do not have a severe scoliosis, do not want to undergo an operation, or are not satisfied with the result of the previous operation. They are looking for body perfection. Before or after their spine surgery, they may continue in their search for a perfect body and seek out surgery for their breasts, lips or nose in a sort of pilgrimage of plastic surgeons. Consequently, we have to respect their experience because their feelings may be very painful and cause anxiety. The asymmetry and the imperfection they see turn into something invalidating to their personal identity. They do not like their physical selves and may believe that because they have scoliosis, nobody will love, appreciate or desire them. With these patients, it is unlikely that surgery will solve the problem. They will constantly find more imperfections in their back, in their shoulders or in another part of their body. Therefore, surgeons and other professionals have to pay close attention to these patients. This is an internal perceptual problem, rather than a physical problem and they need psychological support, such as therapy. Consequently, we have to sharpen our intuition, by giving a searching look to the patients, asking them about previous operations, watching their bodies. Seemingly meaningless details such as the meticulous care of their nails, eyebrows, etc. can give us insight into their level of body perfectionism.

These patients may suffer from a mental disorder, called Body Dysmorphic Disorder.

According to the Diagnostic and Statistical Manual of

Mental Disorders[50], *body dysmorphic disorder* is a diagnosis related to a high-level of distress due to a perceived physical anomaly that people experience in the form of persistent and intrusive thoughts. *Body dysmorphic disorder* can cause one to avoid social situations and intimacy; it can also lead to depression, isolation and potentially suicide[51]. Although *body dysmorphic disorder* affects from 1% to 2% of the general population, being able to recognize this disorder in a patient with idiopathic scoliosis, is of extreme importance for the proper planning of an individualized treatment.

---

50   American Psychiatric Association. Diagnostic and statistical manual of mental disorders (5th ed.; DSM-5). Arlington, VA: American Psychiatric Publishing. 2013

51   Kenny T, Knott L, Cox J. Patient.co.uk. [Internet]. England. [Updated 2017 Feb; cited 2019 Feb]. Available from: http://www.patient.co.uk/health/body-dysmorphic-disorder

### Clinical Case: The Woman with the Pump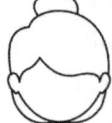

When I met her, she was lying in bed after a second operation for scoliosis. Even if a bit of time has passed since our meeting in hospital, I can remember her face perfectly: her fair complexion, her blue eyes. She was beautiful. She was totally dependent on opiates. She started telling her story and some days later when I visited her again, she told me that she had also had breast and lip operations years before. When I met her, she was taking morphine using a PCA (Patient-Controlled Analgesia) pump because she told me she was suffering a lot: her pain in a scale from 0 to 10 was a 9. I noticed that while she was talking with me, she did not use the pump.

A deep sadness and loneliness invaded me after speaking to her. This woman needed a lot of psychiatric and psychological support. She presented an extreme case of *body dysmorphic disorder* in addition to depression and drug dependence.

## The Embodiment Experience

As professionals in the treatment of patients with idiopathic scoliosis, an important goal of our work is to promote positive body image. We have several tools at our disposal to help the people manage their scoliosis. We have to consider that the perceptive aspect of body image, the 'aesthetic' criteria, is still important, as we live in a visual and narcissistic society, but it is not the only important aspect. Additionally, sight creates distance between people and their body and if it is the only way to approach body image issues there is a risk of *self-objectification*. "To objectify is to make and treat something that is not an object as an object, which can be used, manipulated and controlled and known through its physical properties"[52]. According to theorists Fredrick and Roberts[53], when people self-objectify their bodies, the focus is on how they think the others look at them rather than on how they feel. As a consequence, self-objectification can promote self-surveillance or vigilant body monitoring.

Many times, I have listened to parents say that doing exercises or wearing a brace will allow daughters to be beautiful, to be loved, or to find a boyfriend easily, etc. I have seen patients from different cultural backgrounds whose parents were worried because their daughters might not find a man because of their scoliosis. The body was seen from an observer's perspective, in this case from a would-be boyfriend's eyes.

We have to consider the treatment as an opportunity for enhancing health and inner body equilibrium. We have to be careful when we talk with our patients, trying to widen their embodiment experience and their idea of their own body image.

Is it possible to perceive the body from a different perspective? Piran (2017)[54] defined the concept of embodiment as the experience of body-self integration. She researched the

---

52  Calogero RM. Objectification Theory, Self-Objectification, and Body Image. In: Thomas F. Cash, editor. Encyclopedia of Body Image and Human Appearance, Vol 2. San Diego: Academic Press; 2012. pp. 574–580.
53  Fredrickson B, Roberts T. Objectification theory: Toward understanding women's lived experience and mental health risks. Psychology of Women Quarterly. 1997; 21, 173–206.
54  Piran, N. *Journeys of Embodiment at the Intersection of Body and Culture: The Developmental Theory of Embodiment.* San Diego, CA, US: Elsevier Academic Press. 2017.

construct of the experience of embodiment in women and found the following five dimensions:

1. Body connection and comfort, characterized by feeling "at one" with the body;
2. Agency and functionality, when people feel their bodies physically active;
3. Experience and expression of desire, related to the connection to desire and responding to it coherently;
4. Attuned self-care, in terms of attunement to internal needs (bodily, emotional, relational and existential needs);
5. Inhabiting the body as a subjective site, resisting objectivation.

Positive embodiment is related to experiencing the body as a "comfortable" place from which to connect with the world. It means paying attention to our body from the inside, having consciousness and awareness of its needs and desires. The word consciousness (from Latin: "cum+scire", to know, be conscious) means knowledge. In mindfulness practice, attention is directed into the body as a way of self-knowledge, of information of tension, contractions, tiredness or vitality. Inhabiting our body can be described by a metaphor of a home. As we do with a home, we should clean and adorn the body from the outside, but also experiment with our body by, activate or relax it from the inside. We can take care of it only on the outside or, on the contrary, we can look into its inner depth and neglect its outside layer. So, if it is like a home, a space of support and protection, how do we live in our body?

Moreover, if the body is our home, the vertebral column could be the invisible axis of the home. When I went inside the leaning tower of Pisa, I felt like I was inside a building with scoliosis - it is surely a professional distortion! A spiral staircase goes up the tower from the ground to the terrace on top and looks as though it is a crooked spine. As in the vertebra of a person with scoliosis, each rung of the staircase is slightly tilted and it was fun to see a tilted landscape from the side windows.

In psychology, qualitative tests based on drawings are used to get to know a person, their needs, desires and ways of functioning. One of this is aptly called the House-Tree-Person test[55] as the patient is asked to draw a house, a tree and a person. This test is used to discover more about their personality, self-esteem, body image, etc.

I frequently use the Drawing of the Human Figure[56] in clinical practice as a manner of getting to know people and their embodiment, as well as to use it as a reference when I later interview the patients. I use this test as it provides a lot of information about the way people live their body. Moreover, the results are really indicative when it reveals the patient's omission of certain parts of the body. In a previous research[57], in a sample of 50 adolescent and young patients with IS, 34% (n=17) patients did not draw any facial features. In literature[58], omission has been related to evasiveness or superficiality. When I worked with patients in a group, I asked the patients who drew themselves if something was missing and often they were not able to recognize the missing parts until

---

55  Gordon RM, Rudd-Barnard A. House-Tree-Person Test. In: Kreutzer JS, DeLuca J, Caplan B (eds). Encyclopedia of Clinical Neuropsychology. New York, NY: Springer; 2011

56  Machover K. Personality Projection in the Drawing of the Human Figure. Springfield, IL, US: Charles C. Thomas Publisher; 1949

57  D'Agata E, Rigo M, Pérez-Testor C, Puigví NC, Castellano-Tejedor C. Emotional indicators in young patients with Idiopathic Scoliosis: a study through the drawing of Human Figure. Scoliosis. 2014 Dec 12;9(1):24

58  Hammer EF. Guide for Qualitative Research with the H-T-P. J Gen Psychol. 1954;23(4):489–492.

another patient in the group pointed them out. One young girl who, upon being told of her complete omission of detail, looked at me deeply, connecting, said: "I know why I didn't draw myself inside - it is because I am not personalized". This was the most insightful answer I had ever received. Identity "arises from a feeling of contact with our body"[59] or, as the psychologist Erikson says, *identity is the sense of being at home with his own body*[60].

Here are the drawings of those adolescents representing this lack of identity construction.

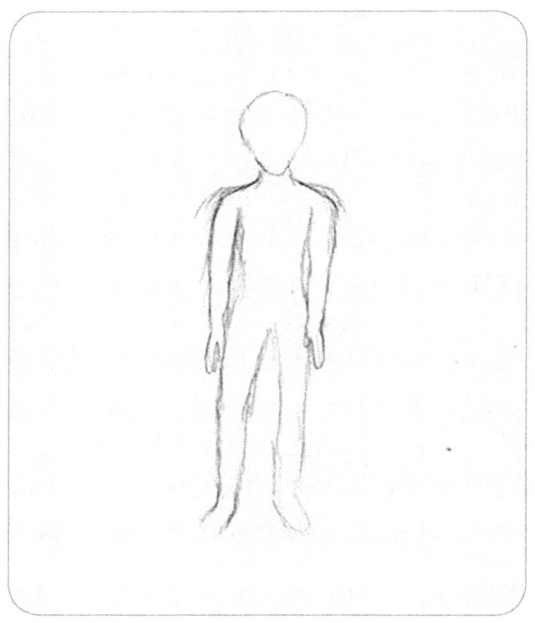

---

59  Ressler A, Kleiman S. Experiential and Somatopsychic Approaches to Body Image Change. In: Thomas F. Cash, editors. Encyclopedia of Body Image and Human Appearance, Vol 2. San Diego: Academic Press; 2012. p. 418–424.
60  Erikson, E. H. Identity: Youth and crisis. New York: W. W. Norton; 1968. p.165

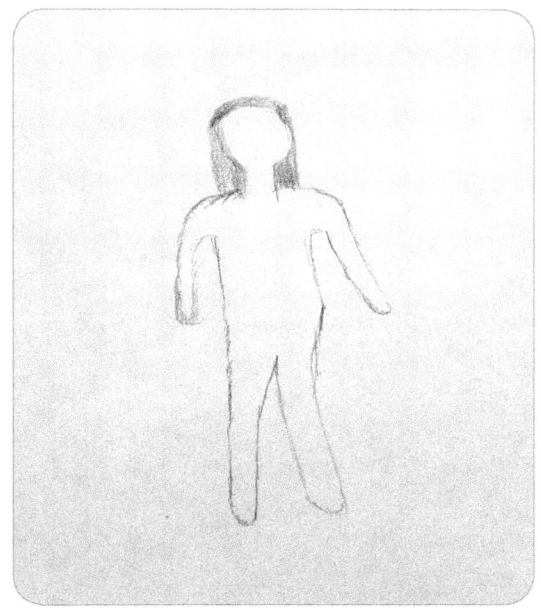

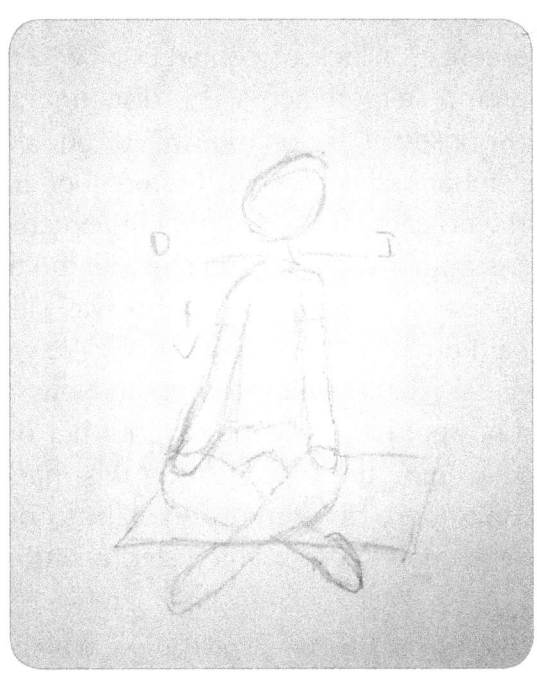

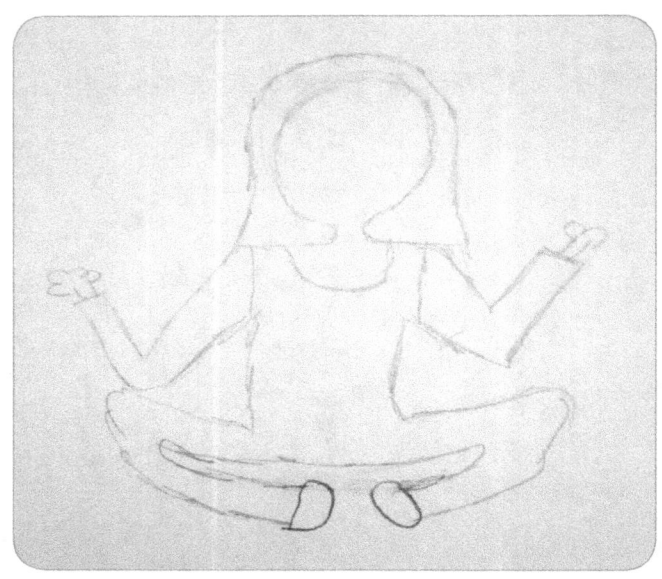

I called these drawings 'ghosts' to define the absence of identifying features of their age, sex, personality, etc. As well, during adolescence, a lack of connection with the self can be a quite common experience[61]. This disconnection can explain their responses of "I don't know" to our questions, as well as their embarrassed silences. I remember, in particular, a Spanish girl who came to the hospital in September. I asked her about her summer vacation and she told me that she had done nothing special. Her mother, who was sitting closely next to her, said angrily: "Nothing special? We went to New York!". It is evident that the mother went to New York, but her daughter did not go; her body moved, but her dull soul did not wake up to enjoy the trip. Hearing this made my heart sink. Stories like these drive me to explain to professionals that these adolescents seem uninterested or indifferent: it is

---

61  Siegel D. Brainstorm: The Power and Purpose of the Teenage Brain. New York: Penguin Group; 2013

not because of their character that events in their lives can be experienced as being "nothing special". They felt into this state and so they can live again and revive their souls: they can reconnect with their vital potential and with their deep inner self.

Walking along the enormous Golden Gate Park in San Francisco, I came across some twisted trees that reminded me of scoliosis again (sorry, I am incurable!). As I previously mentioned, there is another psychological drawing test that consists of drawing a tree as an expression of one's personality.

The tree drawings tell us a lot about people's life, their vitality and perceived emotional and physical strength, as well as their embodiment. In the first drawing below, entitled "The Tree of Colors", the lack of roots converts it into a floating tree, not grounded or belonging to the earth.

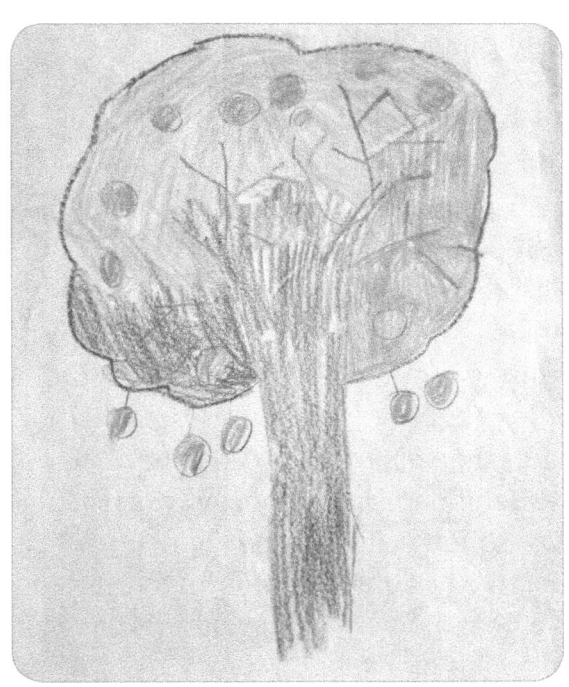

On the contrary, the second tree is big, rooted and structured. It lives in two conditions: the sun and the moon. The boy who drew this tree explained to me that the moon represents the state of exhaustion before sessions, while the sun represents the state of relaxation after sessions.

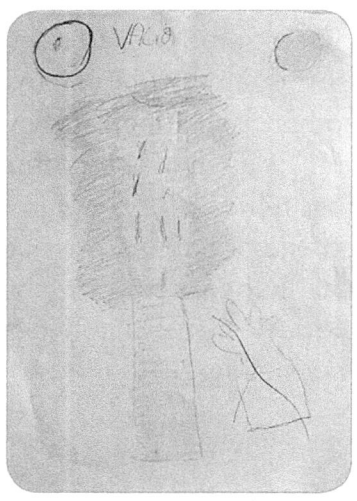

There is also a Japanese story that describes the contrast between the strong, unbending oak and the flexible, twisting bamboo: the trunk of the strong oak in front of the storm tries to resist, but it is so hard that it cannot bend to the winds and at the end it breaks. While the bamboo, which bends with the winds thanks to its flexibility, stays alive. You may have seen some Instagram images of scoliosis columns where it is written: "bent but not broken", associating flexibility and the bending of the spine to the capacity of coping with the storm of life. Behind this metaphor, an existential struggle for life appears. Inspired by this observation, I use a visualization technique that you can also apply in your physical therapy sessions, as a final moment of relaxation. Here is an example of the visualization of a tree.

## ♯1♯ Visualization: My personal Tree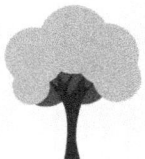

To realize this visualization, the person should be standing, in a comfortable position, keeping their feet in contact with the floor, hips-width apart.

*Flexing the knees a bit, without tension, straightening down the arms, eyes closed or slightly lowered, fixedly gazing towards a spot.*

*First of all, try to enter a state of relaxation, take three deep breaths, lifting the diaphragm to open up the chest and then be aware of the circulation of the air in the body; then feel, from the inside, the feet, legs, hips, front part of the trunk, posterior back, neck, head, arms. Afterwards, try to visualize yourselves as a tree: What is it like?*

*Starting from the bottom, how are its roots? Are they deep or superficial?*

*What about its trunk? Is it big, stable, firm, continuous, uninterrupted... or thin, delicate, ethereal? Is the tree tall or tiny? What kind of leaves does it have? Are they abundant, scarce or are there no leaves? Does the tree have fruits (what kind and color are they)?, etc. Carefully observe its shape, colors and size. In which season of the year does this tree live? Does it bloom in spring? Does it produce fruit in summer? Does it die a little in winter or in autumn? Is it alive? Does its sap circulate internally or does it no longer reach its extremities and is it dying?*

*...*

> ...
> 
> *Slowly, bring your awareness again to your breathing and to the body. Breath in and breath out deeply three times. Taking your time, start moving the body and when you are ready, open your eyes.*
> 
> *At the end, you can draw your tree and/or share your experience.*

## Body postures

In my work as a researcher at a hospital, I used to photograph patients. I realized that most of them had problems with awareness of their posture; when they stood still while waiting for the camera click, their body was oblique with one shoulder higher than the other, their head rotated. In front of a mirror, they could recognize their misaligned posture and correct themselves, but without the visual feedback of a mirror they were not able to do so. When they were lying down, they stayed obliquely misaligned, but they felt as if they were lying straight; they needed posterior control to check their alignment between their feet and their head.

According to a review made by a French group of authors[62], it is likely as not isolated dysfunction at a vestibular level, but rather a disturbance in the multisensory integration of vestibular, visual and somesthetic input which affects an erroneous central representation of verticality and, as a consequence, difficulty of orthostatic postural control. In re-

---

62  Catanzariti JF, Agnani O, Guyot MA, Wlodyka-Demaille S, Khenioui H, Donze C. Does adolescent idiopathic scoliosis relate to vestibular disorders? A systematic review. Ann Phys Rehabil Med. 2014 Aug-Sep;57(6-7):465-79.

cent research,[63] the authors found an erroneous perception of the Gravitational Vertical in patients with right thoracic IS. Furthermore, shoulder obliquity has been considered [64] as a postural deviation associated with IS.

All these postural disorders related to asymmetry, obliquity and verticality can be found, surprisingly, in the patients' drawings. The patients were not aware of the clear asymmetry of the representations in their drawings.

he first drawing below was made by a boy with slight scoliosis; no evident asymmetry was present in his shoulders, although he represented it on an unconscious level, but in a very observable way.

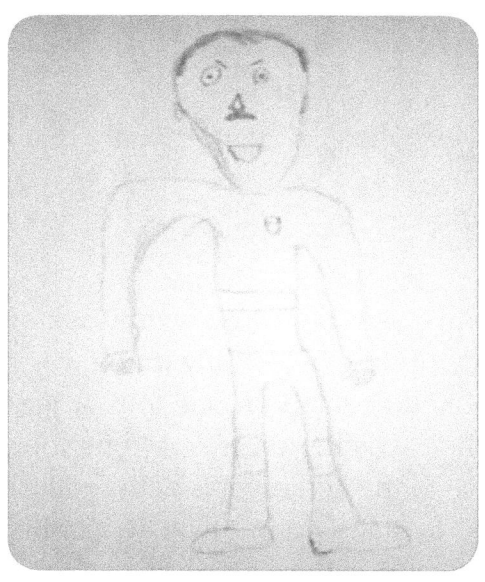

---

63   Le Berre M, Pradeau C, Brouillard A, Coget M, Massot C, Catanzariti JF. Do Adolescents With Idiopathic Scoliosis Have an Erroneous Perception of the Gravitational Vertical? Spine Deform. 2019 Jan;7(1):71-79.
64   Penha PJ, Penha NLJ, De Carvalho BKG, Andrade RM, Schmitt ACB, João SMA. Posture Alignment of Adolescent Idiopathic Scoliosis: Photogrammetry in Scoliosis School Screening. J Manipulative Physiol Ther. 2017 Jul - Aug;40(6):441-451

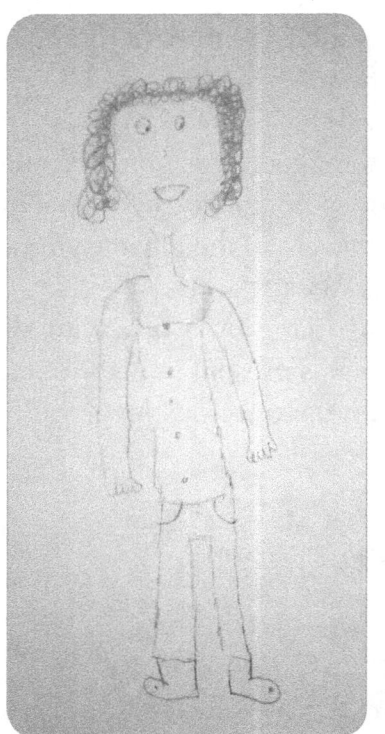 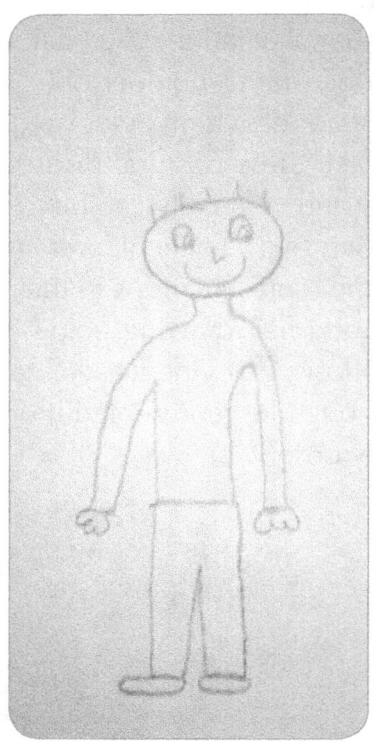

I have always been surprised by the lack of awareness of their own body posture, especially in the way they stand up. Most of them tend to stand on one foot or leg. This foot can change and their weight moves from one foot to another. It is not exclusive to the adolescents with scoliosis, but most of them are used to standing in this way. Furthermore, if they have a solid support at their disposal, such as a wall or a table, they would lean their body on it.

### The Girl with Her Father

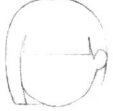

"Lucy" was an adolescent with IS who came to therapy, as she had been suffering from heavy bullying since her childhood. She had scoliosis and was wearing an asymmetrical brace that was quite visible. Her body posture was very impressive: she walked in a such an unbalanced way that she seemed to be limping. When she was waiting for me with her father in the hall, she would stand on one straight leg with all of her weight on her big supportive father. One leg was rooted to the ground while the other one was dangling in the air, as if free of the force of gravity.

"Do you have in mind the sensation of serenity, pleasure and security that gives the power of being supported, the feeling that someone or something supports you? That's what you cannot feel when our misaligned bones do not allow us to rest firmly on the ground"[65]. We may not feel secure by leaning with only one leg on the ground. Our nervous system would be on alert to prevent us from falling and would have to activate a series of compensatory muscles so that we could stay in that position.

*Keep your feet on the ground* in contrast to *have your head in the clouds* are common colloquial expressions present in many languages. They are related to staying in touch

---

65  Puig T, Tolja J:¿Demasiado peso sobre tus espaldas?[Internet]. [Cited 2018 Feb]. Available from: http://www.bodythinking.com/es/salud/demasiado-peso-sobre-tus-espaldas%e2%80%a8/

with reality, to being centered. In Bioenergetics, a method of psychotherapy created by Alexander Lowen, M.D., this concept was developed as "Grounding"; symbolically, it means to stay in touch with reality[66] and to nurture oneself.

The drawing below was made by the girl who defined herself as "un-personalized", one year later she did her first drawing at the end of the course. This time she "personalizes" herself in drawing by including hair and facial features, but ... what happened to her feet?

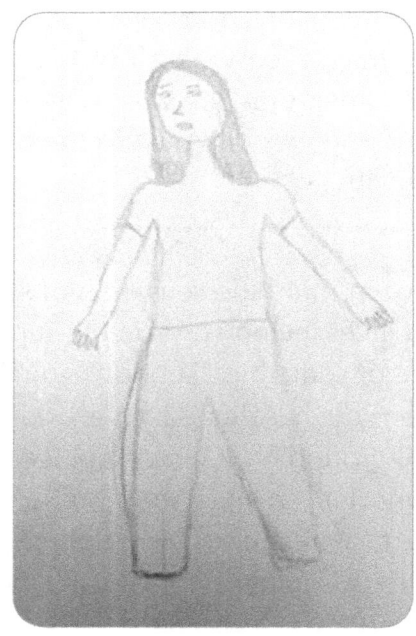

---

66    Ressler A, Kleiman S. Experiential and Somatopsychic Approaches to Body Image Change. In: Thomas F. Cash, editor. Encyclopedia of Body Image and Human Appearance, Vol 2. San Diego: Academic Press; 2012. p. 418–424

## ♯2♯ Playing with Body Posture

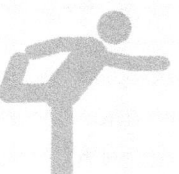

I invite patients to take different postures, apart from self-correction. Maintaining the present posture, exaggerating it or minimizing it, passing from a habitual posture to a self-corrected one in a slow motion, like in a movie; or fast forward, speeding it up, changing velocity of movement. Repeating these movements at different speeds sharpens and widens the patient's sensitivity to a world of perception, emotions and thoughts.

*What is your physical sensation when your posture is not aligned? What happens to your rib cage? To your breathing? How does what you see change when you straighten your head and you see the world from this new perspective?*

Patients can observe their own body postures, listen to their internal breathing and perceive their heart beating. Finally they can make contact with their inner sense of self.

It is important to encourage patients to observe their body with warm attention. Sometimes, patients with scoliosis look towards their body absently or as if to dismiss what they see. Faced with a body failure, people may consider their body as ugly. Teaching them to embrace all parts of their body is a way of taking care of it, not only for finding beauty in their appearance and appreciating themselves from the outside (self-objectivation), but for enhancing their health, inner care and self-esteem.

## Brace: The Challenge of a Crisis

It is known how challenging wearing a brace is for an adolescent, especially at the beginning, for its general difficulty related to breathing, eating, moving, sleeping, sitting, having social relationships, etc.[67] It is a time of crisis and it causes a state of grief: the adolescent loses not only the previous comforts, but also the future ones which they were dreaming of and hoping for related to the world of their peers, social life and events, romance, physical activities and autonomy. As entering adolescent's social life has its own language, its own habits and dress-code, commonly bracing does not fit in this world. As a consequence, over a span of 6 to10 months, initial reactions of isolation, self-marginalization behaviors and denial of the problem are common[68]. Feelings of fear (when looking at the mirror, as if they are carrying a huge weight), anger (towards their parents, the doctor and themselves) and shame (at school, being looked at by friends or classmates in a strange way)[69] can be experienced. After this first period of acute stress, the situation can normalize, although the feeling of discomfort continues in many patients[70].

However, as with any difficulty, bracing is double-sided:

---

[67] Donnelly MJ, Dolan LA, Grande L, Weinstein SL. Patient and parent perspectives on treatment for adolescent idiopathic scoliosis. Iowa Orthop J. 2004;24:76-83.

[68] MacLean WE Jr, Green NE, Pierre CB, Ray DC. Stress and coping with scoliosis: psychological effects on adolescents and their families. J Pediatr Orthop. 1989 May-Jun;9(3):257-61.

[69] Sapountzi-Krepia D, Psychogiou M, Peterson D, Zafiri V, Iordanopoulou E, Michailidou F, Christodoulou A. The experience of brace treatment in children/adolescents with scoliosis. Scoliosis. 2006 May 22;1:8.

[70] Andersen MØ, Andersen GR, Thomsen K, Christensen SB. Early weaning might reduce the psychological strain of Boston bracing: a study of 136 patients with adolescent idiopathic scoliosis at 3.5 years after termination of brace treatment. J Pediatr Orthop B. 2002 Apr;11(2):96-9

it can be a danger or an opportunity. It always depends on the way a person is able to cope with this drastic change. Some coping strategies in case of stress are more useful than others[71]. Those who use an *avoidance style* tend to deny the existence of the problem and then they do not seek help, isolating and escaping from reality: "My scoliosis is not as serious as doctors say", "Wearing a brace is not a problem for me ...". In the beginning, this coping style reduces stress, but as it is only a temporary mental escape from the reality of their situation and not a process of consciousness, it is often a self-trap. The adolescent needs to have the courage to really look at the brace they wear, not to dismiss or avoid it.

Those who use an *approach style* try to face the situation and take action to solve the problem. It can be expressed by asking questions, searching for information, meeting people with a similar experience and trying to deeply understand the problem. In the immediate term, this attitude towards the problem can increase worries and stress. However, the patient can find more effective ways of living with a brace.

## Brace Wearing Preparation

I often say that wearing a brace is like setting out on a new journey or going on a pilgrimage. A few years ago, I went on a pilgrimage on the *Camino de Santiago* and I walked for days on an ancient path taken by many pilgrims in the north of Spain. It was a very rich, personal experience. What allowed me to enjoy the *Camino* was the preparation I took before taking on this endeavor. I spoke with a friend who was a real expert on making the trek. Before leaving, a pilgrim

---

71   Arble E, Arnetz BB. A Model of First-responder Coping: An Approach/Avoidance Bifurcation. Stress Health. 2017 Aug;33(3):223-232.

has to choose a good, comfortable backpack, selecting only essential objects to be put inside for the appropriate weight, to get informed about the websites for the different stages of the trek, to overcome fears and to trust in himself. In fact, you can imagine how hard a long journey on foot can be if the shoes are not suitable - the blisters on your feet can turn it into torture. In the same way, wearing a brace may be a long, unknown and uneasy journey, that can significantly change the traveler, not only in their Cobb degrees, but also in their deep personal growth. To have a good bracing experience, a 'backpack' of essentials and doing all the preparation in terms of gathering information and organizing your life, are indispensable.

**Parents** need to be informed: they need to read the literature on IS and they need to talk with different professionals to fully understand the options and solutions that are available. They need to share the weight of the 'backpack' with their partners otherwise they may suffer from isolation and anxiety from carrying this burden alone. Talking with other parents who are living a similar experience can be a great source of relief and support.

In fact, when I worked with the patients in groups, informal self-help groups of parents would talk together over coffee while waiting for their daughters. They became a group of friends, allies and accomplices, who supported one another. This was thanks to an initial presentation given for the parents where information about scoliosis and the basic rules of the group organization were provided.

If we treat patients individually, we can organize a social day for our patients and their families where they can meet each other. We can help them by organizing icebreaking activities, as outlined below (#3#). They will greatly appreciate it as their need of sharing their experience and finding support from others is very high.

> ### #3# Initial group presentation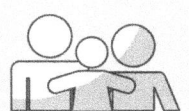
>
> As patients are commonly shy in the beginning, staying with their parents can let them feel a sense of comfort during the first sessions. On the adolescents' side, the presentation consists of introducing their parents to the group, stating their names, ages, professions, and including their hobbies, etc. while parents should introduce their children in the same way. The environment is pleasant and encourages a relaxed way of working together.

While preparing the patient's travel 'backpack,' usually adolescents wear shirts under their brace and buy larger-sized clothes to go over the brace and hide it. Parents and patients have to learn how to take care of the patient's skin, keep its elasticity and moisturize it in pressure areas, checking for sores.

On the other hand, similar to the stages of a journey, it is important to help the adolescents to organize their daily routine and plan weekly activities. As adolescents live an intense school life, marked by homework, essays and exams, it is important to coach them on how to include extra-curricular activities, such as sports and social activities as sleepovers, parties and dinners. Furthermore, it is helpful to organize the time spent without a brace, planning it in advance as a time for celebration or relaxation. Whether it is an hour or a few hours, it is important to enjoy this time and engage in activities that promote self-care such as going to the gym, taking an aromatherapy bath, having a massage, etc.

Finally, friends, classmates, family and relatives can be of a great help to the adolescent, however, at the beginning, they can be seen by the adolescent as a problem. I know patients who never told their classmates about their brace; they made a great effort and it took a lot of energy to dissimulate and camouflage their brace, to appear different from who they were, to control their outfits and their gestures, hiding their condition with shame. Exposing oneself in front of an entire class and explaining scoliosis and its treatment requires a lot of strength and courage. Sometimes, they do not feel ready but, with the help of an adult, they can learn an important life lesson: to cope with shame, to be brave and to be honest and authentic with others.

As professionals, we can give suggestions to our adolescents, for example to talk about the brace progressively with their best friends, then with the teacher and eventually with the whole class.

## Adherence

Sometimes I see patients who collapse passively inside their braces, surrendered. They can develop an acceptance of treatment if we help our patients to deeply understand the functions of the brace.

First of all, doctors should include patients in the discussion and decisions of how the treatment will be carried out. A brace is not an imposition: costs and advantages have to be explained, so that the patients understand and can choose the best option for their health. This gives them an opportunity to 'buy-in' to the treatment and helps them to develop their autonomy[72]. When the patient and his family have "bought into" the idea of wearing a brace, the next step is to go to an orthotist. With the aim of acceptance in mind, the colored catalog created by orthopedic technicians can help adolescents with the transition. In this book the adolescent feels free to choose the graphic designs and colors to be printed in their brace. In the personalization of a brace, the colors they choose can tell us a bit about their personality, their likes, their vitality, their acceptance, and gives them a sense of independence.

---

72   Donnelly MJ, Dolan LA, Grande L, Weinstein SL. Patient and parent perspectives on treatment for adolescent idiopathic scoliosis. Iowa Orthop J. 2004;24:76-83.

## ♯4♯ Initial self-expression: two lists

Ignoring what the adolescents think about a brace is not a good strategy. To create a space where the adolescents can express all their emotions and difficulties related to the brace is important, in order to feel free, to share, to be listened to, to feel supported and to make sense of it all.

The first part of the activity consists in telling or writing all the negative things they think and feel associated to the brace: "it is uncomfortable, it makes me feel embarrassed, it limits my movements, etc." We or the patient can write it on a piece of paper. I call this the "junk list". After that, we reflect on the points in favor of wearing the brace through a "gratitude list". This part can be hard - sometimes we have to encourage them to find positive aspects and look towards the outcomes and reasons for wearing it. This could have to do with its functionality, a new experience, etc., but they always come around at the end.

In this way, we have the opportunity to integrate both aspects of reality: negative and positive and then to have a more realistic perspective of what wearing a brace means to them.

To help in the process of transition and adapting to the brace and taking the example of the metaphor of a journey, you can reinforce the previous work with the below activity.

## ♯5♯ Passport

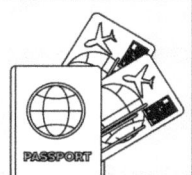

This work consists of two parts: the first one made with creative and manual work; the second part is social. After the previous self-expression work, teenagers try to define in more depth what wearing a brace means for them. They can cut out a piece of cardboard and write the brace information as if it were a passport or an identity card: the brace's name, the brace's "date of birth", its qualities, colors and so on. The adolescents are asked to find a name for their braces because they have to spend a lot of time with it. We can ask our patient to draw a picture of the brace, as if it were a photo to stick in its ID card or passport.

The social part of this exercise is presenting the brace to friends; on the Internet, there are many creative ideas on how to organize a sleepover or a party to introduce a brace with its name and attributes (for example in the blog https://www.bracingforscoliosus.org).

With the *Passport* activity, we can get in touch with many of the adolescent's beliefs about a brace. A patient in the hospital where I worked, for example, named her brace Torture, another Turtle (because it protected him as a little house), etc. About the written qualities of the brace, the most common are painful, tough, ugly, protective, and faithful. There are patients who believe that the pain caused by a brace is normal. Once a girl, who was asked to write daily the sensations caused by her brace, wrote a diary that was really a pain journal. Every day she felt pain, she woke up in pain, she went to sleep with pain, she could not sleep because of the pain... every day for six long months.

When dealing with teenagers, we should not take anything for granted. All these activities and exercises give us an opportunity to explore their personal experience and their beliefs, to explain the difference between suffering from discomfort and suffering from pain. In fact, as there are some patients who are constantly complaining, there are still others who do not even report any discomfort, although they have severe skin reactions or sores, as they consider it normal.

## I don't want this stuff!!

Not every teenager is willing to pay the price of wearing a brace, for different reasons. Sometimes, parents may not understand the use of a brace, considering it obsolete, underestimating the risks of the progression of the curve, etc. and not supporting the adolescent in this type of treatment. Sometimes, refusing a brace can be a form of gaining independence in their adolescent development towards autonomy. The most rebellious adolescents may reject the treatment[73].

When a teenager rejects a brace, it is common to hear desperate parents asking: "How can you not understand? It is good for you, otherwise the curve will advance and your back would be more crooked for your whole life!". An expression of shock and astonishment is drawn on their faces. The lack of compliance could be considered a risk behavior. Maturation-

---

[73] Rivett L, Stewart A, Potterton J. The effect of compliance to a Rigo System Cheneau brace and a specific exercise programme on idiopathic scoliosis curvature: a comparative study: SOSORT 2014 award winner. Scoliosis. 2014 May 30;9:5.

al neurological changes predispose the adolescent towards risk behaviors, expressed as consumption of alcohol, drugs, etc. This choice would be influenced by a state of incomplete maturation of the adolescent brain, called *Transitional Age Brain*[74]. It is characterized by a discrepancy in maturation between the already developed structures, the subcortical (limbic) area and the immature areas of frontal cortex, which is responsible for planning, forecasting the consequences of actions, and satisfaction. The astonished questioning parents could find a possible answer in a neurobiological issue related to the neuro-plasticity of the evolving adolescent brain. This may explain why adolescents find it difficult to understand the consequences of not wearing the brace and to plan and organize the hours of treatment in their life.

## Traces of brace

The experience of the treatment and of scoliosis do not end when the doctor says: "it is time to remove the brace." Some patients have difficulties in giving it up. Due to its closeness to the body, a brace becomes assimilated into the cerebral representation of the body schema as an extension of the body, such as a t-shirt or a pair of trousers[75]. Here is, the experience of a reader of my blog who wore the brace when she attended high school: "(the brace) *was already part of me. In such a way, at the end of the treatment, I missed it*". At the end of the treatment, a body memory as a "trace" of the

---

74  Konrad K, Firk C, Uhlhaas PJ. Brain development during adolescence: neuroscientific insights into this developmental period. Dtsch Arztebl Int. 2013 Jun;110(25):425-31.
75  Carlson TA, Alvarez G, Wu DA, Verstraten FA. Rapid assimilation of external objects into the body schema. Psychol Sci. 2010 Jul;21(7):1000-5.

experience remains; some patients report the sensation of not feeling supported and sometimes they feel the need to sleep with it again.

Contrarily, with reference to the entire treatment, sometimes a patient tries to exclude this part of their history, avoiding talking about it, inhibiting his memory and thereby denying it. However, sometimes spontaneous thoughts, images, dreams of wearing a brace and painful emotions may appear to the patient. For this reason, I suggest an end-of-treatment activity to help patients say farewell to the brace.

---

### ♯6♯ Bye-bye brace!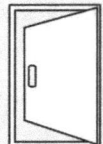

I ask patients to write a letter or a simple message when leaving the brace. As at the beginning, I ask them to write about the negative experiences of living with a brace, as well as the opportunities the brace gave them. This is a ritual of farewell. At the end, patients can bury the letter, burn it, or cut it into many small pieces and throw them into the sea, into the river or scatter them to the wind.

---

The conclusion of the treatment can be a great opportunity to end the process well. It is not only related to the brace itself, but also to scoliosis, to the patients' spine and to their entire body image.

Enjoy Life with Idiopathic Scoliosis during Adolescence

In synthesis, the main points of this chapter are summarized below.

## The 10 Key Points of Chapter 3

1. Body Image is a multidimensional concept that includes perception aspects and attitudes (thoughts, feelings and behaviors) towards the body. Body Image applied to Idiopathic Scoliosis comprises the mental representation of the trunk size and its related attitudes.
2. Not all the patients with Idiopathic Scoliosis suffer from a problematic body image. The degree of dissatisfaction falls on a continuum from low to intense dissatisfaction that could be psychopathological, as in *body dysmorphic disorder* (BDD). BDD is a rare psychiatric condition that affects from 1% to 2% of general population; it is caused by an inner perceptual distortion and not be resolved by physical treatments.
3. As professionals of scoliosis, we can promote a healthy body image, avoiding the experience of self- objectification, that is, treating the body as an object, seen from an observer's perspective.
4. The experience of Embodiment is more related to the feel of the body, to a successful body-self integration. It includes five dimensions: Body Connection, Functionality, Expression of Desire, Self-Care, and Inhabiting the Body.
5. The adolescents' search of identity, disconnection and difficulty with their embodiment could be common experiences. *#1# My personal tree* is a visualization exercise to help patients promote a Body Connection.

6. Patients with IS seem to present problems with verticality and shoulder obliquity control. ♯2♯ *Playing with postures* is a proposed activity to exaggerate or minimize the pattern of postures, playing also with the rhythm, in order to widen the patient's sensitivity to an aligned body posture and body feelings.
7. Brace experience is usually a crisis that challenges the patient's and his family's lives. It requires a period of adaptation and is a double-sided coin: a danger and/or an opportunity for a new life experience. As a journey, it requires preparation. Informal support groups between parents can have advantages. ♯3♯ *Initial group presentation* is a suggested activity to introduce parents and patients to one another so they may find support and understanding of their experience.
8. To enhance adherence, it is advisable that patients have the power to choose their treatments, once pros and cons have been explained. ♯4♯ *Self-expression* is an activity aimed at helping patients to express feelings, thoughts and behaviors towards a brace, first with a *junk list* and later with a *gratitude list*. ♯5♯ *Passport* is a creative activity to personalize the treatment, in order to redefine the relationship of the adolescents and their brace.
9. Problems with adherence could be attempts at the patient's autonomy which can result in immature risk behavior, as explained by the Transitional Age Brain theory.
10. Once a brace has been removed, traces of it could be present in patient's body schema, dreams and memories. Some patients miss their brace. ♯6♯ *Bye-bye brace* is a way of saying goodbye to the brace and gaining closure at the end of the process, defining the negative and pos-

itive experiences that the brace gave them, similar to the *junk and gratitude* lists at the beginning of treatment (♯4♯ *Self-expression)*, closing the circle.

# Chapter 4
## Emotions

*But feelings can't be ignored,
no matter how unjust or ungrateful they seem.*
—**Anne Frank**

*Dance, dance, dance
otherwise you are lost.*
–**Pina Bausch**

## Introduction

The purpose of this chapter is not to write an extensive review about emotions at a theoretical level, since there is a large number of specific handbooks on this topic. Instead, the aim of this chapter is to give a few wide brushstrokes about the most common emotions awoken by scoliosis and braces, such as shame, fear, anger[76] and sadness. Additionally, as emotions are universal internal phenomena, I hope you can find the theories and activities useful for your personal life as well.

Emotions are 'complex functional wholes' that organize

---

76   Sapountzi-Krepia D, Psychogiou M, Peterson D, Zafiri V, Iordanopoulou E, Michailidou F, Christodoulou A. The experience of brace treatment in children/adolescents with scoliosis. Scoliosis. 2006 May 22;1:8.

our thoughts and actions[77]. They present specific patterns of physiological activity and characteristic facial, postural and vocal expressions. In fact, emotions are not only a phenomenon within the brain, they are also made by body responses as "changes in heart rate, blood pressure, skin conductance, and respiration. Among these physiological responses, respiration has a unique relationship to emotion. While the primary role of respiration concerns metabolism and homeostasis, emotions such as disgust, anger, and happiness also influence respiratory activities"[78].

Emotions have a clear adaptive biological aim: our survival. For example, a lion that surprises us activates an intense response of fear and a series of complex psychophysiological reactions that allow us to flee and save our skin.

Furthermore, emotions are also signals for ourselves and for others. They are a type of communication: inner signals to be perceived[79]. An emotion is a message for ourselves and for others.

Sometimes, a person, experimenting an emotion, such as sadness, anger or shame, has the desire to immediately release it. In fact, there are many emotions that are uncomfortable to live with depending on their intensity.

What is our relationship with emotions?

Honestly, sometimes, it is not easy to know the answer to this question. As a psychologist and psychotherapist with personal experience in the management of emotions, I confess that I sometimes try to ignore them. At times, I wait for

---

[77] Barish, K. Emotions in Child Psychotherapy: An Integrative Framework. New York: Oxford University Press; 2009. p11-14

[78] Masaoka Y, Izumizaki M, Homma I. Where is the rhythm generator for emotional breathing? Prog Brain Res. 2014;209:367-77.

[79] Barish, K. Emotions in Child Psychotherapy: An Integrative Framework. New York: Oxford University Press; 2009. p11-14

them to magically leave, like unwanted guests knocking on my door, hoping they get tired of ringing the bell. However, the emotion stubbornly remains where it is until I recognize it, open the door and listen to its message. It produces specific sensations in the body, as if it were a "squatter" that takes over my inner territory according to a precise map of invasion, affecting some organs, causing dreams, thoughts, stomach pain, etc.

Emotions visit everyone. They universally challenge us to create space and time in our lives for them and to let them express themselves. "If they do not express themselves, they rot internally," said Victor Orive, one of my professors. "Emotions are like water... don't allow them to stagnate or they will start to smell bad. They have to flow like a river and carry us with them."

People make an effort to modulate their positive or negative emotions and their expression. These processes have been labelled Emotion Regulation (ER). They are considered to be extremely important for the process of normal development. Maladaptive regulation strategies are predictors of psychological disorders, poor academic performance, low social adjustment, and altered interpersonal functioning[80].

According to Bradley[81], there are two types of maladaptive strategies: the first focuses on a restricted emotional expression and avoidance of the emotion with strategies such as panic, *self-criticism*, rumination, social inhibition, interpersonal isolation, concentration difficulties and attention prob-

---

80   López-Pérez B, Gummerum M, Wilson E, Dellaria G. Studying Children's Intrapersonal Emotion Regulation Strategies from the Process Model of Emotion Regulation. J Genet Psychol. 2017 Mar-Apr;178(2):73-88.
81   Bradley B, DeFife JA, Guarnaccia C, et al. Emotion dysregulation and negative affect: association with psychiatric symptoms. J Clin Psychiatry. 2011;72(5):685-91.

lems; the second focuses on heightened emotionality with typical behavior such as aggression, alcohol and substance abuse, eating disorder, self-harm and suicidality. These strategies represent, in part, the failures of emotion management and "efforts to escape emotions experienced as overwhelming or intolerable" (Bradley et al. 2011).

## *I don't know*

When I was 14 years old, my drama teacher asked everybody at the end of the class: "What are you thinking about during the class? What emotions have arisen today?". When my turn arrived, I had no answers and I stuttered an embarrassing: "I don't know." I would really have liked to give an answer, but I didn't have any idea...none at all. No emotions came to me. Like in a cyclic history, now I am the one who asks to these adolescents: "How are you?" usually they answer: "OK" or "fine"; it seems impossible to get something more out of them. I feel the difficulty of reaching these children deeply.

A difficulty in identifying and describing feelings is associated with a pubertal maturation in girls[82]. This difficulty is called *alexithymia*. Alexithymia also includes poor imagination and a concrete way of thinking[83]. In the book *Brainstorm*[84], Siegel wrote that emotional disconnection is common in adolescent people. Results demonstrated that alexithymia is related to the use of the strategy of suppres-

---

82   Van der Cruijsen R, Murphy J, Bird G. Alexithymic traits can explain the association between puberty and symptoms of depression and anxiety in adolescent females. PLoS One. 2019 Jan 16;14(1):e0210519.
83   Karukivi M, Saarijärvi S. Development of alexithymic personality features. World J Psychiatry. 2014 Dec 22; 4(4):91–102.
84   Siegel D. Brainstorm: The Power and Purpose of the Teenage Brain. New York: Penguin Group; 2013

sion of emotions and in particular to difficulties in verbalizing emotions[85].

Misterska et al.[86] found a high level of *self-criticism* in a sample of non-operated patients with IS compared with a healthy control group, but they did not assess the presence of any psychopathological disorders. As we saw in the previous subchapter, self-criticism belongs to the strategies of Emotional Regulation (1st group) based on the restriction of emotional expression. In another article [87], the same group of researchers did not find a significantly different rate of alexithymia in girls with IS compared to a healthy group. However, they found a lower level of alexithymia in adolescents with IS who participated in sports activities. Finally, we [88] have assessed personality traits in a sample of patients and found the common trait introversion, regardless of their Cobb Angle.

In my experience, likely influenced by the cultural and social background where I am immersed, I have found that the most common profile of adolescents with scoliosis is that they are good students, self-demanding and responsible patients. Parents are usually deeply satisfied with their school performance. Adolescents try to adhere to adults' expecta-

---

85    Laloyaux J, Fantini C, Lemaire M, Luminet O, Larøi F. Evidence of Contrasting Patterns for Suppression and Reappraisal Emotion Regulation Strategies in Alexithymia. J Nerv Ment Dis. 2015 Sep;203(9):709-17.

86    Misterska E, Glowacki M, Harasymczuk J. Personality characteristics of females with adolescent idiopathic scoliosis after brace or surgical treatment compared to healthy controls. Med Sci Monit. 2010 Dec;16(12):CR606-15.

87    Misterska E, Glowacki M, Adamczyk K, Glowacki J, Harasymczuk J. A longitudinal study of alexithymia in relation to physical activity in adolescent females with scoliosis subjected to Cheneau brace treatment: preliminary report. Spine. 2014 Aug 1;39(17):E1026-34.

88    D'Agata E, Sánchez-Raya J, Bagó J. Introversion, the prevalent trait of adolescents with idiopathic scoliosis: an observational study. Scoliosis Spinal Disord. 2017 Nov 8;12:27.

tions, but this behavior can hinder their personal process of finding themselves.

In the hospital, we suggest that parents encourage their children to try expressive activities such as drama, dance, painting, drawing, singing, playing an instrument, etc. These activities allow personal self-expression, an exposure to others, an outward movement in opposition to the tendency of withdraw and isolation into oneself.

Furthermore, for many years, I accompanied a treatment group that had weekly physiotherapy sessions. Thanks to the permission of the responsible doctor, with the physiotherapist in charge, we offered an integrated physiotherapeutic treatment: my focus was aimed at encouraging personal expression and self-knowledge.

I was touched by the great sensitivity of these patients - when being helped to connect with their emotions, they expressed creative ideas and very deep, noble feelings. They really suffered and struggled in school: school was a source of great pressure to them. I remember a patient who had to come for individual therapy on Friday afternoons, so as not to miss study hours during the week.

At the beginning, the disconnection of these adolescents affected me a lot, but nowadays I realize that it is common in adolescents as well as in adults. It is not healthy, but it is frequent. There is too much information coming from the outside world and it can interfere in us receiving the not-so-easy information from our emotions that come from within. If we do not give space to what is inside us, listening to our inner world, we end up filled up with images and external noises, feeling empty, or worried and sad.

## #1# How are you? The game of the cards

This exercise is really simple and especially works well in the beginning of treatment as an icebreaker, in a group or individually. To get to know a teenager, I usually use images. I have collected a lot of postcards or fliers of events, shows, concerts, etc. I show them the cards and then ask the adolescents to choose the one they like. Then the patients have to explain the reason they chose this card and any associations related to the image. It usually works, it is fun, and the conversation flows easily.

The exercises below helps to progress toward inner connection.

## #2# Breathing in pairs

As we see in the Introduction of this Chapter, breathing is closely related to emotions: "respiration has a unique relation to emotion" [89] Working with the breath can be of great interest with these patients, as it helps them to connect with emotions, but also relaxes their nervous system.

...

---

89  Masaoka Y, Izumizaki M, Homma I. Where is the rhythm generator for emotional breathing? Prog Brain Res. 2014;209:367-77.

> ...
>
> In fact, breathing patterns have also effects on the cardiovascular and autonomic function, shifting towards parasympathetic dominance[90].
>
> If you work in group, you can manage the exercise as a paired activity, or you can work individually with your patient. One patient lies down on the back, relaxing with closed eyes. You or the other partners sit nearby, observing the breathing style of their patient lying down: the manner in which the person breathes, how long each phase lasts (breathing in/out), any pauses, possible variations of the wave of respiration over time. Then the observers ask them to breath slowly, using controlled, slow breathing. "Six breaths per minute, causes blood pulse fluctuations to synchronize with the heart beat rhythm"[91], relaxing the person.
>
> At the end it would be interesting to listen to the person talk about their emotional state and finally the partner can give them feedback of their observation.

At present, different programs of stress reduction through mindfulness have been performed for adolescent students and in the literature, results are controversial. Even if it seemed not to be useful to improving emotional regulation [92], the pro-

---

90   Russo MA, Santarelli DM, O'Rourke D. The physiological effects of slow breathing in the healthy human. Breathe (Sheff). 2017;13(4):298-309.
91   Russo MA, Santarelli DM, O'Rourke D. The physiological effects of slow breathing in the healthy human. Breathe (Sheff). 2017;13(4):298-309.
92   Kaunhoven RJ, Dorjee D. How does mindfulness modulate self-regulation in pre-adolescent children? An integrative neurocognitive review. Neurosci Biobehav Rev. 2017 Mar;74(Pt A):163-184.

gram was assessed to be effective to reduce depression [93], stress and anxiety [94].

### ♯3♯ *Mindsight* to create the connection

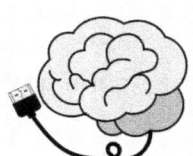

This exercise is aimed at giving space to the inner world, at listening to it and making the person aware of their physical sensations, inner thoughts, and feelings. It comes from the book *Brainstorm*, by Dan Siegel[95]. Siegel calls it *Mindsight* exercise. It is easy to manage. For this exercise we need a calm and quiet place, with cell phones turned off and computers disconnected. First, with closed eyes, focusing the attention on **physical** sensation, the patients are asked to connect with the tension in their muscles, their heart beat, their breathing and their whole body. Next, they have to focus their attention on the **images** in their mind, their memories or hopes for the future. Then, they concentrate their attention on their **feelings**, which could be related to inner thoughts, perceptions or memories. And lastly, they are asked to become aware of their **thoughts**, that could come to them as an inner voice or a sensation.

---

93  Chi X, Bo A, Liu T, Zhang P, Chi I. Effects of Mindfulness-Based Stress Reduction on Depression in Adolescents and Young Adults: A Systematic Review and Meta-Analysis. Front Psychol. 2018 Jun 21;9:1034
94  Langer ÁI, Schmidt C, Aguilar-Parra JM, Cid C, Magni A. Effects of a mindfulness intervention in Chilean high schoolers. Rev Med Chil. 2017 Apr;145(4):476-482.
95  Siegel D. Brainstorm: The Power and Purpose of the Teenage Brain. New York: Penguin Group; 2013

## Sadness

*"When I make the first brace for a patient, he usually cries"*: a German orthopedic technician once told me.

Sadness is an emotion generated by the loss of someone or something we deeply value, or the lack of sense of control or of achieving a goal, according to Paul Ekman (1999)[96]. Sadness affects personal behavior with a tendency to self-marginalize and impacts us physically through posture, with a typical protraction of the shoulders[97]. Scoliosis and brace treatment belong in such way to the loss of control, health and freedom. When it happens, it is sometimes uncomfortable for professionals to stay close to the embarrassing tears of a silent adolescent.

If we put ourselves in their shoes, we can understand their tears. *Crying is a normal way of venting. If you try to hold it in, you will feel much worse.* Allowing our patients to express their sadness through crying can give them a real release, more than reassuring them or trying to repress them by saying: *"Don't cry, you are too old to cry!"* Sadness is connected to social support. Giving them the permission to cry, to feel weak, but supported, helps them to accept the situation. "People around us can, in some cases, soften the blow" [98] By allowing them to cry you are saying: *"Here you are not alone; we will make the journey together. I will help you as much as I can. Ask me for what you need. I will not let you be alone."*

I have met a lot of sad adolescents; the reasons for their

---

96   Ekman P. Basic emotions. In Dalgleish T, Power M J, editors. Handbook of Cognition and Emotion. New York, NY: Wiley; 1999. p 45–60.
97   Rosário JL, Diógenes MS, Mattei R, Leite JR. Can sadness alter posture? J Bodyw Mov Ther. 2013 Jul;17(3):328-31
98   Aaron Ben-Ze'ev. Subtlety of Emotions. Cambridge, MA: MIT Press; 2000. p.112

sorrow were different, for example they may have conflict with their parents or difficulty managing their life.

In the past, I worked with a group of adolescents with scoliosis that really impressed me. I call them "The Group of Heroes".

### The Group of Heroes

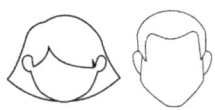

I remember this group, made up of 5 adolescents, who kept their eyes down, immersed in a cold silence. They were united by the same issue: the death of a family member. I did not know this until I found a drawing from a girl in the group. At first, I could not see anything special, except that she had drawn a person, as you can see in the drawing below. I thought that maybe it was herself, her back turned, standing in front of a tree with a big eye and an important element of decoration, asymmetrically expressed on the right and left sides.

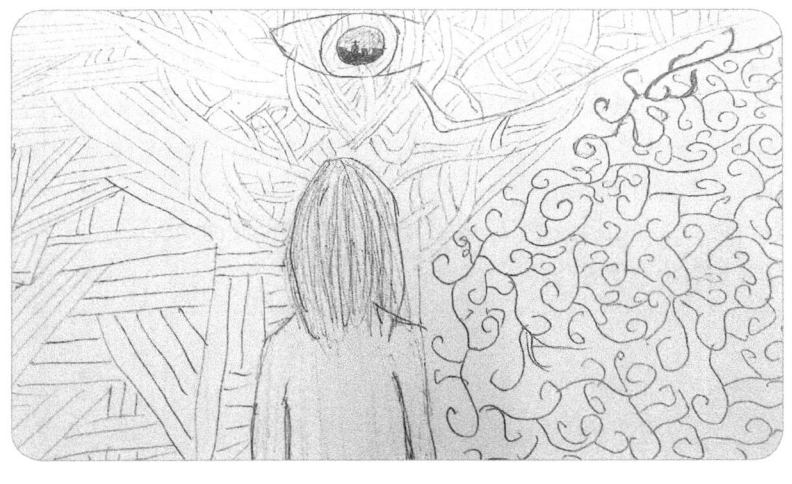

However, looking at it carefully, I saw something that made me tremble ... the eye had a cross inside.

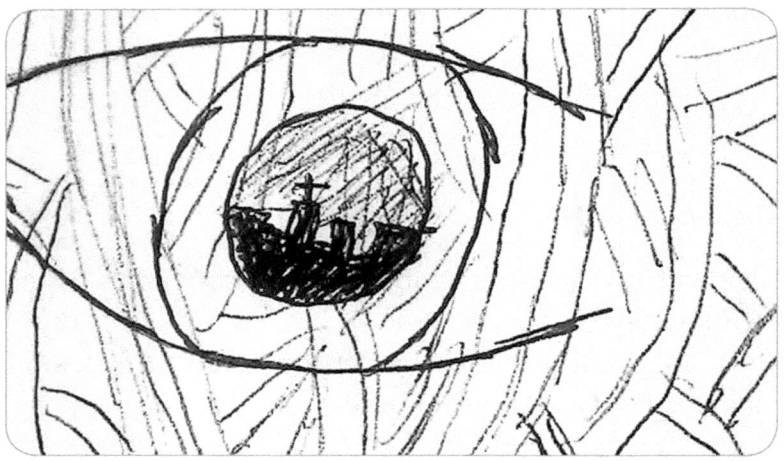

She explained it was a church and that her father had died two years before. She loved him a lot. She was still grieving and possibly depressed. Sadness is temporary and differs from depression, which is "an affective disorder generated by the perception we cannot cope with the loss" [99]. The most therapeutic action came from a shy boy in the group who said to her: "I understand," explaining that his father had left his whole family when he was a child. For him, it was as if the father was dead: he never saw him again.

Empathy is all here: *I lived the same experience - you are not alone.*

---

99  Barish, K. Emotions in Child Psychotherapy: An Integrative Framework. New York: Oxford University Press; *2009*. p11-14

> The other three people did not speak but, later I knew, they were also burdened with experiences related to death. It was unforgettable, so many "deaths" experienced by such young lives! I sincerely still thank them immensely for their trust and courage to break the wall of silence and suffering where they had taken refuge and to connect in such a deep and intimate way.

Accepting sadness with self-compassion can help people adjust to their new circumstances.

However, in 2018 during the SOSORT Meeting, a surgeon claimed he did not want to ask his patients too many questions as Pandora's box could be opened and uncontrollable "monsters" might get out. That surgeon was right in some ways - the sadness of others and their traumatic experience may be scary to us. Sometimes these "monsters" are really frightening. As a professional, when you recognize the existence of an issue in your patient and have problems managing it, asking for a consultation with a therapist or a psychologist is a *professional ethical duty*. Sorrow does not disappear by itself if it is deep: it needs warmth and it needs to be brought to light. Seeking help from a therapist or a psychologist can help your patients to learn emotional self-regulation.

## Shame

A lot of braced patients suffer from shame. Shame is related to the fear of other people's judgment. *What would they say if they discovered my brace?! What do they think when they see my asymmetrical waist?!* There are girls who are victims of their own secret and try to hide their braces or body;

hiding it causes them a great deal of tension: they often avoid physical contact with others and control the way they dress, their posture, their hair, they etc.

Shame is a universal emotion evoked by a sensation of personal failure or inadequacy, especially in public exposure[100]. It includes a range of subjective experiences ranging from embarrassment to a painful feeling of humiliation. Situations related to exclusion or being laughed by others at can be really uncomfortable and can enhance their feeling of shame. The characteristic action associated to shame is concealment. If the emotion lasts over time, then it can severely limit personal growth.

Patients could think: *How can I date anyone with this brace?* They evade eye contact from others, hide themselves in the background. They want an invisible existence.

Contrarily, pride is the opposite of shame: it is associated with outward movement, to exhibit or show oneself to others. Pride is expansive while shame contracts body, thoughts and imagination[101].

Shame involves the whole self. Shapiro and Powers wrote[102]: "the most natural response to the experience of shame (to hide) is the most toxic, whereas the least automatic or natural (to expose) is the most healing". This means that it is healthier to communicate the existence of the brace to friends and classmates from the beginning. However, it does not often come naturally to do so.

---

100  Barish, K. Emotions in Child Psychotherapy: An Integrative Framework. New York: Oxford University Press; *2009.*
101  Barish, K. Emotions in Child Psychotherapy: An Integrative Framework. New York: Oxford University Press; *2009.* p11-14
102  Shapiro E, Powers T. Shame and the paradox of group therapy. In: Dearing R, Tangney JP, editors. Shame in the therapy hour. New York: Hardcore; 2011.

What can we do to help manage their shame? Shapiro and Powers (2011) gave us some advice in the psychotherapeutic setting that can be adapted for the brace treatment:

- Simply talking about the shame provoked by the brace and scoliosis in a safe context can reduce the pain of shame.
- Being empathic with the client's discomfort, normalizing their desire to hide; telling them about a time in our own lives where we have experienced shame can humanize their experience.
- To regulate shame, it could be useful to ask the patient to imagine themselves giving advice to a real or imaginary friend wearing a brace.
- To empower patients, we should encourage them not to be ashamed, to hold their head high. This gives patients a sense of dignity instead of shame. Sometimes, humor can help to empower them by creating a playful environment, to evoke laughter instead of crying. There are a lot of useful suggestions online, such as organizing a party to present the brace, making a cake decorated with reference to scoliosis, etc. (https://www.bracingforscoliosus.org).

Marianne Williamson expressed shame and fear versus feelings of empowerment in her poem [103]. I consider it a rich source of inspiration:

*Our deepest fear is not that we are inadequate.*
*Our deepest fear is that we are powerful beyond measure.*
*It is our light, not our darkness*
*that most frightens us.*

*We ask ourselves*
*Who am I to be brilliant, gorgeous, talented, fabulous?*
*Actually, who are you not to be?*
*You are a child of God.*

*Your playing small*
*does not serve the world.*
*There is nothing enlightened about shrinking*
*so that other people won't feel insecure around you.*

*We are all meant to shine,*
*as children do.*
*We were born to make manifest*
*the glory of God that is within us.*

*It's not just in some of us;*
*it's in everyone.*

*And as we let our own light shine,*
*we unconsciously give other people permission to do the same.*
*As we are liberated from our own fear,*
*our presence automatically liberates others.*

---

103  Willamson M. A Return To Love. New York: Harper Collins; 1992. p. 190-191

## #4# Roleplaying: How can you introduce the brace to your classmates?

To overcome shame is a heroic act - to face reality and to show what is hidden can end the secrets.

Role-playing is a tool of training relational behaviors, where people as actors rehearse situations in preparation for their future performance, as it happens on a stage. This gives them the opportunity to improve social abilities, to reflect on their difficulties, and to find strategies in order to cope with reality.

In this case, a roleplaying activity could be practiced to prepare for the time when they introduce their brace to their friends or classmates.

As physiotherapists, brace technicians and psychologists, we should first prepare the communication with our patient, asking: *How would you tell your class?* It is possible they have told their best friends about the brace, but if not we can suggest that they confide first in their closest friends, as they can be a great source of support and understanding.

We can then play different roles with our patient, simulating different settings, from the easiest to the most difficult: we can act as one of their friends or a teacher, even an unpleasant classmate, or an entire group of people or class.

...

> ...
>
> As a consequence, our patients will test and improve their communication skills in different situations, gaining confidence in preparing to reveal the brace to others. We can start with a simple question: *What would you say to me if I was your...?*
>
> If our patients are really stuck and do not know what to say, we start off by playing their role while they act as the audience. They may even be critical in their role, releasing their fears about what people might say and giving us the opportunity to show them how to handle the most difficult interactions. This gives them the opportunity to integrate new personal scripts while they learn new vocabulary and abilities. Then, we should change the roles and have them play themselves so they can practice these new tools they have learned.

## Fear

*To improve adherence, is it good to threaten the patient by showing them the consequences of the progression of scoliosis and that they might need an operation or their shoulder could become disfigured?* I have received this question many times from professionals having difficulties with adherence from their patients.

Fear is one of the basic emotions, characterized by a highly negative effect and physiological excitation; it appears in situations of danger and prepares the organism to face the danger or to escape[104]. Fear is an emotion with a specific facial expression called wide-eyed morphology[105]. According to literature, fearful expressions mimic a babyish face with large eyes and high forehead. The aim of presenting this expression is socially communicating helplessness to stimulate human support. It is opposite to the expression of anger with narrowed eyes, communicating maturity and dominance.

The information about a possible threatening stimulus is quickly scanned in the amygdala, our primitive subcortical brain, and once the threat is detected, various types of defensive responses, for example the activation of our sympathetic system, are triggered[106]. Patients wearing a brace because they are scared of surgery or women afraid of the progression of their scoliosis during menopause can be very different cases where fear controls their lives.

Fear and anxiety are related, but there are different factors involved. Fear is generated when a concrete threat is detected: a patient has to wear a brace or has to be operated on. Anxiety may appear without the presence of an actual threat, as they prepare for unexpected danger: the patient has to be treated in case of scoliosis progression. Worry is the prototypical example of anxiety. When worrying, a person thinks about negative things and possible negative outcomes. The opposite experience of fear and anxiety is the feeling of safety and security[107].

---

104 Barish, K. Emotions in Child Psychotherapy: An Integrative Framework. New York: Oxford University Press; 2009. p11-14
105 Sacco D. Fear expression: Function and Form (p.69-71) in Gervais AD (edit). Psychology of fear. New York: Nova Science Publishers; 2011.
106 Muris, P. Normal and Abnormal Fear and Anxiety in Children and Adolescents. San Diego, CA, US: Elsevier; 2007. p. 2.
107 Barish, K. Emotions in Child Psychotherapy: An Integrative Framework. New York: Oxford University Press; 2009. p11-14

The strategy of threatening a patient describing the possible consequences is not appropriate as it depends on the patient's fear level and coping mechanisms. Furthermore, it is not ethical due to the difficulty in predicting the progression of scoliosis[108]. It is also a very different thing to threaten patients rather than informing them and their families about the possible evolution of scoliosis.

In the case of fearful patients, and more often their parents (as just said in chapter 2), it is important to remember that they can evoke all the possible catastrophic interpretations related to the situation and the threat could cause them to have unnecessarily high levels of anxiety.

Moreover, patients' most common fears are usually related to being excluded by their group of friends at school. We can counter this by helping them to explore: What is their group of friends like? How is their relationship with their peers? Have they experienced incidence of bullying in the past?

These patients can change and become resilient. Resilient adolescents in general adapt well in the face of risk and adversity, showing higher levels of global self-worth and psychological well- being[109]. How can we help our scared patients to become resilient adolescents? They have to live an experience of feeling safe associated with brace treatment.

The activity below can be really useful to help scared or anxious patients, patients who have to undergo surgery, and even to help stressed professionals to relax themselves.

---

108 Donnelly MJ, Dolan LA, Grande L, Weinstein SL. Patient and parent perspectives on treatment for adolescent idiopathic scoliosis. Iowa Orthop J. 2004;24:76-83.
109 Muris, P. Normal and Abnormal Fear and Anxiety in Children and Adolescents. San Diego, CA, US: Elsevier; 2007.p. 101

## ♯5♯ Visualization of a safe place

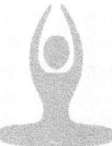

(This is mostly directed to psychologists, as it belongs to psychotherapists' or coaches' training.)

The therapist asks the clients to find a good body posture (lying or sitting, as they prefer), with closed eyes, in order to relax and to connect to their breathing. After that, they invite the patients to imagine a place where they can feel safe. The place can be real or imaginary. It could be part of nature (on a beach or in a forest) or somewhere else. The therapist guides the patients through the exploration of that place, asking them to be aware of all the stimuli they may find: Visual (What can you see?), Auditory (Are there any sounds?), Olfactory (Can you smell any scents?), Tactile (Can you touch something nearby?) Maintaining the patient in this state of relaxation, the therapist asks: How do you feel there?

If the imagery gives the patients comfortable, pleasant sensations, the therapist invites them to linger some time there, to enjoy the sensation, breathing there. Contact with a safe place allows the reduction of muscular tension, deep breathing and pleasant feelings. The therapist can invite the patients to go into this place whenever they need to, or whenever they have fear or anxiety. This image can be a really powerful tool for the patient to manage challenges in their life.

...

> However, sometimes, the patients can encounter anxious or scary images. For example, pre-surgical patients can see strange and unsafe places - sometimes they are cold and isolated places. In this case, the therapist can invite them to change or improve the image: Which details would you like to add to your image? Can you make it brighter there?
>
> After that, the therapist kindly asks the patients to find a path to come back to reality, breathing deeply and moving different parts of the body. When they have slowly re-awakened the body and are coming back to reality, they can open their eyes. Lastly, they can draw the safe place as a way to imprint it into their memory.
>
> ...

## Anger

*"At first, I was angry with my parents, with the doctor, with myself"; "During the first days I was very angry and I was behaving hostile towards everybody"*.[110] These are two statements about the feeling of anger at the beginning of a brace treatment in adolescents with IS; adults can also feel angry about their appearance or their pain and the usual question, "Why me?" frequently arises.

Anger is an emotion evoked when we are exposed to frustration or to a goal blocking event, physical injury or emotion-

---

110 Sapountzi-Krepia D, Psychogiou M, Peterson D, Zafiri V, Iordanopoulou E, Michailidou F, Christodoulou A. The experience of brace treatment in children/adolescents with scoliosis. Scoliosis. 2006 May 22;1:8.

al pain. A restriction of freedom of movement can also be a source of anger, as observed from the age of 3 or 4 months[111]. This is interesting because a brace can be felt as a limitation of free movement.

As a reaction to anger our muscles tense up while respiration and heart beat accelerate, blood pressure increases and the whole body becomes ready to attack[112].

The basic circuitry of anger is subcortical, relating to the limbic area, where amygdala plays a key role in its modulation. There, our primitive and immediate reactions take place, while integrating fibers with a calming action lie in the prefrontal cortex. Subcortical limbic areas are more active in adolescents than in children and adults because during adolescence the prefrontal area is under reconstruction. For this reason, adolescence is a stage of emotional intensity [113].

Tomaszewski and Janowska (2012)[114] assessed a sample of girls who had to undergo surgery. They presented *contained anger*, that is, they found difficulty in expressing their rage. Almost the entire sample presented a style of internal anger, meaning that patients could not express their anger related to this difficult situation in which they were living.

In my experience with adolescents with scoliosis, I met patients with a need to express their anger towards their classmates or teachers; their exams or their homework were frequent objects of anger. Sometimes they asked me for help

---

111   Barish, Kenneth. Emotions in Child Psychotherapy : An Integrative Framework, Oxford University Press; 2009, p. 23.
112   Pahlavan, F. Multiple Facets of Anger: Getting Mad or Restoring Justice? Hauppauge, New York: Nova Science Publishers; 2011.
113   Siegel D. Brainstorm: The Power and Purpose of the Teenage Brain. New York: Penguin Group; 2013.
114   Tomaszewski R, Janowska M. Psychological aspects of scoliosis surgery in children. Stud Health Technol Inform. 2012;176:428-32.

if they needed to defend themselves from being bullied at school or to put limits on others. I remember shy girls who asked me if they could shout, to speak up and express their inner tension.

Self-regulation is also important for anger. Listening attentively to patients while they are expressing anger towards school, the brace or their parents is a good way to help them liberate their inner tension. Siegel (2013) stated the importance of naming emotions to master them: it helps to calm the inner raging sea as well as to integrate it at a cortical level.

 In synthesis, the main points of this chapter are summarized below.

## The 10 Key Points of Chapter 4

1. Emotions are "complex functional wholes" that organize our thoughts and actions, with specific patterns of physiological activity (heart rate, blood pressure, skin conductance, breathing).
2. Emotions have two clear aims: our biological survival and communication with ourselves and the others.
3. Emotion Regulation (ER) is a process to modulate positive or negative emotions and their expression.
4. Difficulty in identifying and describing feelings is common among adolescents. ♯1♯ *How are you? The game of the cards,* ♯2♯ *Breathing in pairs* and ♯3♯ *Mindsight* are activities to help patients connect with their internal emotional world.
5. The most common emotions awoken by scoliosis and braces are shame, fear, anger and sadness.
6. Sadness is generated by the loss of something that is considered worthy. Scoliosis and the brace may represent a loss of control, health and freedom.
7. Instead of saying *Don't cry, you are old to cry,* give the patient the permission to cry: *Crying is a normal vent. If you try to keep it in, you will feel worse. Here you are not alone; I understand you.*
8. Shame is evoked by a sensation of personal failure or inadequacy, especially in public exposure. The behavior

associated to shame is hiding in the background, with the desire to be invisible. #4# *Roleplaying: How do you introduce a brace to your classmates?* is an activity to cope with shame in the school context.

9. Fear appears in situations of danger and prepares the organism to face the danger or to escape. The opposite experience of fear and anxiety is the feeling of security. #5# *Visualization of a safe place* is a psychological technique used to promote an inner feeling of safety.

10. Anger is evoked when we are exposed to frustration or to a goal blocking event. Regulating the expression of anger is important: naming it in order to master it and to integrate it at a cortical level. Additionally, being listened to by a reliable person can be helpful.

# Chapter 5
## Mind

*To be a person is to have a story to tell*
**–Isak Dinesen**

*Wayfarer, the only way*
*is your footprints and no other.*
*Wayfarer, there is no way.*
*Make your way by going farther.*
**–Antonio Machado**

## The ESSENCE of Adolescence

Parents sometimes say: *They will never wear the brace, they are at that difficult age; they are at an awkward age, you know. I have to control them and make them wear the brace all the time and remind them: put on the brace!; I have to learn all the exercises, so they can do them at home.*

    Adolescence is usually considered a hard time as one is under the effect of a hormonal storm, the adolescent "goes crazy" and is still immature and emotionally uncontrolled, thinking irrationally. Adults have to wait out the storm to get a break; living together, they have to try to survive as best they can. Books for parents such as *"Help, I have a teenager!"*

were popular in the past, stressing the negative view on this period in life.

However, recently, these beliefs have been considered false myths thanks to the latest studies in neuroscience through neuroimaging techniques. Furthermore, these beliefs could be serious obstacles to the complete development of adolescents and also to compliance in the treatment of scoliosis. They can function as a self-fulfilling prophecy as well as a *Pygmalion effect:* when the expectations about people are so powerful that they are able to affect their performance (and not only at school).

Daniel Siegel[115] writes that, thanks to brain changes, four qualities represent the ESSENCE (acronym for the four features) of adolescence: **Emotional Spark**, referring to the intensity of inner sensations, exuberance and vitality at this age; **Social Engagement**, related to the increased importance of social life and connections with peers; **Novelty seeking**, meaning a search for new experiences, new inputs to stimulate senses, emotions, thoughts and body, associated to the need of rewards and to changes in the dopamine circuits in the brain; **Creative Exploration**, linked to abstract and divergent thinking that allows adolescents to solve problems in non-conventional and sometimes revolutionary ways.

Nowadays, adolescence is considered as a phase full of possibilities, a "workshop" with possible different results (D'Avenia)[116]. Rather than making an effort to 'survive' this phase, adolescence is a period that should be lived well, because there are all the conditions to reach fullness, to real-

---

115 Siegel D. Brainstorm: The Power and Purpose of the Teenage Brain. New York: Penguin Group; 2013.
116 D'Avenia A. L'adolescenza non è una malattia [Video on the Internet]. 2014, May 7. Available from https://www.youtube.com/watch?-v=uW_Osb9QJwI&t=67s

ize one's complete potential (Siegel, 2014). If the adolescents achieve it, they can arrive at their personal self-realization. This meaning is explained also by its ancient etymology: the word *adolescence* comes from Indo-European, where the root "*ol*" means "all" (as in the word "holism") and adolescence is a movement towards fullness.

So, adolescents have to be seen and treated not as immature and lazy people, but as people growing with a lot of energy and potential. They are able to do incredible things, such as opposing to a Nazi German regimen as the young Scholl siblings did, or sailing around the world alone as 17-year-old Laura Dekker[117] did in more recent years.

If we consider them as young people able to do extraordinary things, the beliefs about patients' adherence to treatment could also change.

## Adults and adolescents

Recent studies in neuroscience[118] about the adolescent brain, called *Transitional Age Brain,* explains that the adolescent brain is in a period of extreme plasticity: experiences from the environment have the power to influence, divert, enhance and promote the journey of their life. An adolescent brain goes through a process of complete reorganization that consists of "pruning down" the existing neurons and also of the myelination of the remaining neurons[119]. The pruning

---

117    Dekker L. Laura Dekker. [Internet]; 2019 [cited Feb 2019]. Available from: http://www.lauradekker.nl/
118    Konrad K, Firk C, Uhlhaas PJ. Brain development during adolescence: neuroscientific insights into this developmental period. Dtsch Arztebl Int. 2013 Jun;110(25):425-31.
119    Spear LP. Adolescent neurodevelopment. J Adolesc Health. 2013 Feb;52(2 Suppl 2):S7-13.

process means that the abundance of the neural connection obtained during childhood is reduced. As in the process of pruning a garden, all the synapses that 'failed' are lost because of the pruning process. Siegel explains that this process is determined genetically, but also by experience. If the synaptic circuit was not used, it would be pruned. This means that there is a time to cultivate passions and ability, before the pruning process. The pruning process may also be intensified because of stress. Moreover, the new connections are covered by myelin sheaths to speed communication between different parts of the brain. For this reason, focusing the adolescents' attention exclusively on their treatment, on wearing the brace, on their exercises and medical visits, could be seriously diminishing for their life learning, blocking their development.

The adolescent lives in a transformative period. He is like a plant that needs a good quality soil. As adults, we can contribute to enrich this "soil". As professionals of scoliosis, we can offer worthy experiences to our teenage patients. Sometimes, parents do not agree with their children's decision and behave in a reactive way, with anger or fear. Parents that live a constant battle in their house over the brace and treatment, go through difficulty and pain with their teenagers, without good results.

Adolescents need the adults' *presence* rather than their control or criticism, even though parents may think that it is for their own good. *Presence* is related to being receptive, open to what is happening, listening and tuning to their teenager. Additionally, presence creates trust in the relationship (Siegel, 2014).

Furthermore, while adolescents create distance from their parents, the presence of other adults (Supportive Non-Parental Adults) as well coaches, teachers, mentors, tutors, etc. determines the improvement of their self-esteem and reduction of risk-behavior (use of drugs, sexual activity, etc.)[120]. As professionals (physical therapists, orthopedist technicians, doctors, and psychologists), we can also function as Supportive Non-Parental Adults to support them with their emotional difficulties and to reduce their behavioral problems.[121] The benefit is reciprocal. In fact, adolescents and adults have opposite tendencies: adolescents want to create a new world while adults want things to continue as usual (Siegel, 2014). Staying in contact with the new generation helps us keep ourselves alive. In fact, the brain does not only change during adolescence, but throughout our life span. Siegel wrote in his book that the four features characterizing the ESSSENCE of the adolescence are also applicable to adult life; adolescents bring energy to our lives, allowing our brains to grow. In fact, as adults we need the Emotional Spark otherwise we get annoyed or depressed in our mundane routines; we need to be Socially interconnected instead of feeling alone and isolated, to make new friends, to stay in contact with different people; to seek Novelty and creatively explore, otherwise we die under the burden of the repetition. Staying in contact with adolescents gives us the opportunity to maintain contact with the future, with the evolution of mankind. We discover hidden powers of the adolescent's mind, connecting us with

---

120 Yu MVB, Deutsch NL, Futch Ehrlich VA, Arbeit MR, Johnson HE, Melton TN. "It's like all of his attention is on you": A mixed methods examination of attachment, supportive nonparental youth-adult relationships, and self-esteem during adolescence. J Community Psychol. 2019 Mar;47(2):414-434.
121 Sterrett EM, Jones DJ, McKee LG, Kincaid C. Supportive non-parental adults and adolescent psychosocial functioning: using social support as a theoretical framework. Am J Community Psychol. 2011 Dec;48(3-4):284-95.

dynamism and opening us up to novelty, livening us up with their laughter. To prevent depression, rigidity, or falling into routine, it is healthy to nurture our inner adolescent mind.

**Let me to tell you a story**

Daniel Taylor (Ph.D., Emory University) wrote[122] we are the product of the stories we have heard. We were born into stories, they nourish and guide us lifelong. Our great storytellers are family, school and culture. Far from being simple entertainment, the act of storytelling is an answer to the existential question: *Who am I?*

I reflected about the stories patients hear about scoliosis: a mysterious rotation that may be treated with a brace and exercises or surgery. And sometimes, sadness seems appealing, while faith and hope seem far away. Facebook pages used as discussion forums by patients with IS frequently exhibit pessimism[123]. Sad stories limit inner strength.

My aim is to promote adolescents' personal power, to alter negative beliefs about patients with scoliosis and their identities and to push them towards life and exploration. Taylor (2005) affirmed that healthy stories are crucial to make life worthy and diseased stories can be replaced. With the aim of taking advantage of the enormous power of tales, I started searching for stories, myths and legends about scoliosis, humps, deformities, listening to other perspectives, building

---

122   Taylor D. Tell Me a Story: The Life-Shaping Power of Our Stories. St. Paul, MN: Bog Walk Press; 2005
123   Glinkowski W, Agaciak A, Kister A, Glinkowska B, Pulaski K. Analysis of posts about scoliosis by patients on Social media and networks. In SOSORT. XIII International Meeting; 2018 Apr 19-21. Dubrovnik: SOSORT; [cited 2019 Jan 2019]; p.53. Available from: https://www.sosort.mobi/pdf/SOSORT%202018%20Book%20of%20Abstracts.PDF

up creative and positive images about scoliosis. Born from an ancestral need of human beings to give meaning to our complex reality, ancient myths, fables and tales were constructed using the evocative power of words and their symbology in order to connect with the universal social imaginary of mankind.

To my surprise and delight, as an example of empowerment and benefit, I found out two beautiful tales. The first one is the story of two hunchbacks. It is well-known in Italy (Italo Calvino wrote about it in his Collection of Folktales[124]), in Spain (in the Basque Country[125]) and in the British Isles[126].

---

124  Calvino I (1956). Fiabe italiane. Gli struzzi n. 24. Torino: Einaudi; 1956.
125  Xabier Susperregi. Cuentos Vascos- Los dos Jorobados. País Vasco: Biblioteca de las Grandes Naciones; 2017[cited 2018 Jun]. Available from: https://es.calameo.com/books/004654285f7343df86954
126  The Two Hunchbacks and the Walnut Tree. [cited 2018 Jun]. Available from: https://www.jesterbear.com/Aradia/TwoHunchbacks.html

## #1# The story of the two Hunchbacks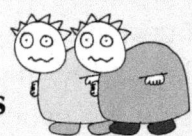

The tale is about the story of two brothers, both with humps. The younger of them decides to undertake a journey to look for fortune and leaves the elder one at home. At night he finds shelter in a walnut tree and there he observes a coven of singing witches. He decides to intervene, adding a verse to their song, an action that completely changes the fate of his life: the grateful witches take his hump away. Happy, he returns home and tells his brother what happened. The elder brother starts the journey immediately, finds the tree witches, observes the coven at night, listens to the song ... and adds his verse. But unexpectedly he provokes the anger of the witches who do not appreciate his addition to their song. The witches decide to punish him by adding the hump of the younger brother. He sadly goes back home with two humps.

This story has many versions, but the general meaning is maintained in all of them. It presents almost all the features of ESSENCE of the adolescence. The young brother starts his journey, leaves the known (the comfortable zone) to find fortune, boosted by Novelty seeking. The journey is related to transformation and self-realization. So, the young brother is a brave man. Furthermore, he is able to engage in Creative Exploration: he thinks of a new verse for the song, using his divergent thinking and the witches reward his efforts. He comes back happily with an Emotional Spark. Whereas, the journey of the elder brother is totally different because it is a copy: he follows the footsteps of his younger brother and there are no risks, the way has been carved out for him. At the end, he is punished by the witches because of his lack of an original search and the absence of risk.

I liked asking the adolescents with IS their personal understanding and meaning of this tale. It was a way to enter their delicate world. Which character do they identify with? Why?

I have often seen adherent patients with their brace looking like zombies, anesthetized and sad. I was surprised by their angelic faces with their trunks collapsed into the brace: their bodies surrendered and fallen inward, deflated in their own vitality.

In my personal experience, I have seen a large number of "good children" in medical consultations, adolescents who make many sacrifices in their life: brilliant students or national champions in some sports discipline. Sometimes, I asked myself if they behave as the younger or the elder brother, searching for themselves or following other people's voices. The search of the true self goes beyond the path drawn by parents or teachers; it is intimate and personal and needs serious and focused intention to realize it.

Living with scoliosis and a brace does not exclude the ESSENCE of the adolescence: not to be stuck to the brace but to search for their own passions, the emotional spark and to experience the flow. The psychologist Csíkszentmihály[127] said when people are in a state of "flow", they immerse themselves totally in the activity, they do not get tired, their energy

---

127 Csikszentmihalyi M, Lebuda I. A Window Into the Bright Side of Psychology: Interview With Mihaly Csikszentmihalyi. Eur J Psychol. 2017;13(4):810-821.

is focused and they live with feelings of happiness, freedom, creativity and joy. No brace can distract from the search of flow experience and of ESSENCE.

The story of the teenagers is not written yet: a teenager's life is like a blank piece of paper - they create their own story, they are the heroes of their own life.

I remember a patient who said that she loved theater, but of course as a hobby, not as a job for her future. Theater was her passion but it was not a serious profession, according to her parents. This voice comes from fear, not from an internal vibration and vitality. I was reminded of the words of another girl: "I like dancing but I have to swim because of my scoliosis"; another 13-year-old girl told me: "I hate going to English class after school, but I have to do it for my curriculum vitae".

For this reason, at the beginning of my course, I prepare an activity to help them express their hobbies, likes and passions, defining who they are.

## #2# The poster
(individual or group activity)

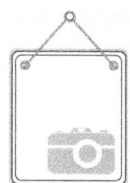

I invite patients to create a poster of their own life, cutting out magazine or newspaper images they like, about hobbies, interests, etc. and then sticks them all on a collage. Each poster is a possibility for them to start thinking about what they like, what they look for; and for us, it is a way to get to know their human side. If we work in group, it is interesting to see how the teenagers connect with each other, because they find similarities in each other. For example, those that have put dogs on their poster have a love for animals in common. The most frequent pictures that appear are handsome boys, makeup, traveling themes, animals, etc. This is a simple way to start a connection, overcoming fears, shyness and break down the wall of "I don't know" that I usually hear as an answer to "what do you like to do?". We can also accompany the activity with classical music, to help them concentrate in a pleasant way. Pleasure is another element we have to bring into the activities. Considering the seriousness of their lives, the common great self-discipline and self-demanding style, it is really healthy to create a warm and cozy environment, where creativity, connection and peace can be encouraged. They are essential ingredients.

## A hunchback God

The second story comes from the legends of the Navajo and Hopi Indian tribes: it is the story of Kokopelli, a hunchback god who plays the flute.

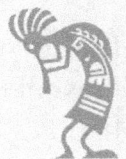

### #3# The story of Kokopelli

This god is a storyteller and a merchant. In his hump he carries his merchandise: feathers, shells, precious stones and seeds. As he is the god of spring, traveling from one village to another, he sows all the seeds he contains in his hump on the ground and so the earth is filled with flowers and plants. The sun appears and the snow melts. The birds sing happily and all the creatures stop to listen to his songs and music. In his hump there are all the musical notes which have not been played yet, all the songs which have not been sung and the stories which have not been heard. On his hump, Kokopelli carries unborn children and distributes them to women. His "hump" is the place of Creativity.

He is a traveler. When he arrives at a village, men and women celebrate him, lighting bonfires, singing and dancing around the fire. He is also a joker and a trickster god, who does not follow the rules, brings gifts and has magical and healing powers. In other mythologies he is comparable to Hermes or Mercury, or to another Italian hunchback, *Gobbo*[128], the spirit of good luck, abundance

---

128 The ABC of Arabia [Internet]; [cited 2019 Feb]. Available from: https://www.jesterbear.com/Aradia/abc.html

> ...
> and fertility. In Italian, in fact, *Gobbo* means Hunchback. In ancient times, people thought that touching the hump of a hunchback would bring them good luck.

Kokopelli has the Emotional Spark necessary to travel and to create art and life; although he is a solitary traveler, he is Socially Engaged with the people he meets in the villages; his journey is an expression of Novelty Seeking and his hunched back is a symbol of Creative Exploration. In conclusion, Kokopelli embodies the ESSENCE of adolescence. A good question to ask is: *How is Kokopelli expressed in our lives?*

With adolescents, the effect of listening to the story of this god usually, at first, evokes reactions of surprise and astonishment and then gets them to become open to the dimension of Creative Exploration. These tales invert the common thinking about the negativity of scoliosis through an identification process. As Kokopelli himself is creative, the tale triggers a direct access to the internal and personal "Volcano". As I was born in a city at the foot of Mount Etna, the highest volcano in Italy, I had the experience of listening to its tremendous roar coming from its bowels. A Volcano and a Hump are powerful images representing places where Creativity and energy are stored.

Myths are ways of communication of meaning since a meaningless experience cannot be understood or lived. This is of great importance especially in our field, as scoliosis is idiopathic, that is, patients do not know where it comes from, it does not have a clear source. Some patients see genetics as the answer (having had a mother or an aunt with scoliosis), others find a different reason for their scoliosis. All of them need to explain it and we do not currently have scientific answers. Because of this need, I have encouraged patients to create and express their personal and narrated sense of their own scoliosis. However, not everyone is ready to enter this dimension of Creative thinking; there can be blocks impeding their creativity and personal connection. These people should not be forced, because it means that it is not time for them to make sense of it yet. But for those who can, they can write their own tales in a surprising way.

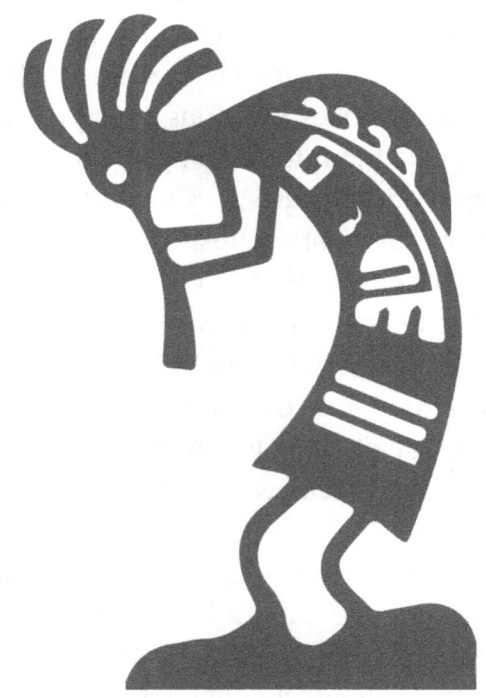

## ♯4♯ Creative scoliosis

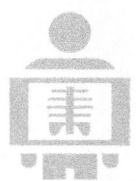

After telling the story of Kokopelli, I show people their own X-rays in order to see the pattern of their scoliosis. In an attentive atmosphere of silence and concentration, with classical music in the background, I first help the patients to listen to their body, to sit comfortably in a chair, both feet resting on the ground (rooting down), paying attention to breathing, and observing the presence of thoughts, emotions, posture, etc. Then, I give each patient a piece of mud or simply a pencil and paper. And I ask them to shape the clay according to their own spine, if they want, they can do this with their eyes closed. Or they can simply draw or can use other recycled materials. I explain that the time they spend, the care they devote and the details they put into their spine represent an act of love toward their spine.

When they have finished, I ask them to touch their sculpture with their fingers. To activate imagination, entering the world of fantasy and creativity, I tell them that their fingers are transformed into ears, listening to the story the clay tells them.

When they finish, I invite them to write the story about their spine, without censorship, without paying attention to spelling or punctuation.

...

...

In my experience, there were a lot of teenagers who looked at me with surprise: they had no idea what to write about, they looked at each other and laughed. So, I told them if they had difficulty writing, they could just write a title instead of the entire story. They always ended up explaining their experience.

For me it was really interesting to listen to them. Many beliefs came out with reference to this back that has been curved: some felt responsible for how badly they treated it by carrying heavy backpacks, others told me about how they felt different to have it.

Each person was respected for their ability to go deeper, or to maintain on the surface.

This voice that the patients "hear" from their fingers touching their clay figure back and writing on paper is an inspired story that they, at first, may not understand. Sometimes, later, they can make a bridge between the story and their biography. I felt very grateful for the trust of all my patients who have allowed me to work with these stories.

## Tales

Cyrulnik Boris is a neurologist and a psychiatrist, who saved himself from detention and Nazi capture with his parents by hiding when he was 6 years old. He wrote[129] that every story is a way to become free. It is a reconciliation with his own life. Communicating our story to others allows us to modify our story. The possibility of making our own story is a central element of resilience. The story is about giving a shape to an image, repairing it, giving coherence to events or healing an unjust emotional or physical wound.

The stories that teenagers tell are often incredible. Inspired by Kokopelli, they talk about long journeys, distant places and archetypal images such as princesses and wise old men. The most significative stories were written in a few minutes, without too much thinking, in a flow experience, as if they 'received enlightenment'. To me these stories are sensitive material, made of the same material as dreams.

The following stories are from teenage patients.

**The wise man with the rod** story was told by a 16-year-old girl with lumbar scoliosis, still being treated with a brace.

*Once upon a time there was a man who visited all the towns and had a very long rod with an ending curve. This man helped anyone who had a problem, whether it was about money or health. By moving his rod a little, he worked miracles. Once a woman who had a disease asked for help, and he cured her. On another occasion, a boy, who had lost a leg, came to him, and he gave it back just by moving that crooked rod. For all the miracles that this man performed, he received nothing in return.*

---

129 Cyrulnik B. Talking of Love on the Edge of a Precipice. London: Allen Lane; *2007*.

*One cold night the wise man was walking through a town when he met a beggar. He was wearing ragged clothes and he was very thin, he seemed to be on the verge of dying. The wise man knew that it would take many miracles to heal that man. But he helped him, gave him fortune, clothes and health, and the beggar soon recovered completely. But nobody knew that every time the wise man moved the rod, a part of him died. Little by little the wise man was consumed. The truth is that he had already lived well for a long time, and he thought it was enough, and he knew that others also deserved an opportunity in their lives.*

**Dune** *was the story by a 16-year-old boy at the end of his pubertal development, with severe stabilized scoliosis, who was never treated with a brace.*

*An old man climbed onto his camel, left his village and travelled for a long time among the dunes without knowing where he was or what his destiny was. The dunes were getting bigger and on several occasions he was forced to take refuge from the storms among his belongings. He struggled to stay alive through the cold nights and not to get dehydrated during the scorching days. One day, in broad daylight, he fell off his camel, exhausted by the lack of water.*

*Days later, he woke up in an unknown house in a big city where they did not speak his language. He ended up staying there and started his own family with the Turkish prince, and with the passing of time he became a king.*

**Columneti** *was the story written by a 10-year-old girl with slight scoliosis and at the time she was not treated with a brace.*

*Once upon a time, there was a column called Columneti and all her classmates mocked her because she was crooked.*

*One day Columneti went to the doctor who told her that she had to put on a brace. Columneti wore the brace for two years until she got the column straight and now none of her classmates make fun of her anymore.*

Two years after she had written this tale, I was present when the doctor prescribed her a brace, as she had intuitively foreseen in her story.

This last story is from a 15-year-old boy, with mild scoliosis: *"She is 15 years old, she is curved and she is yellow"*. You can see his drawing below.

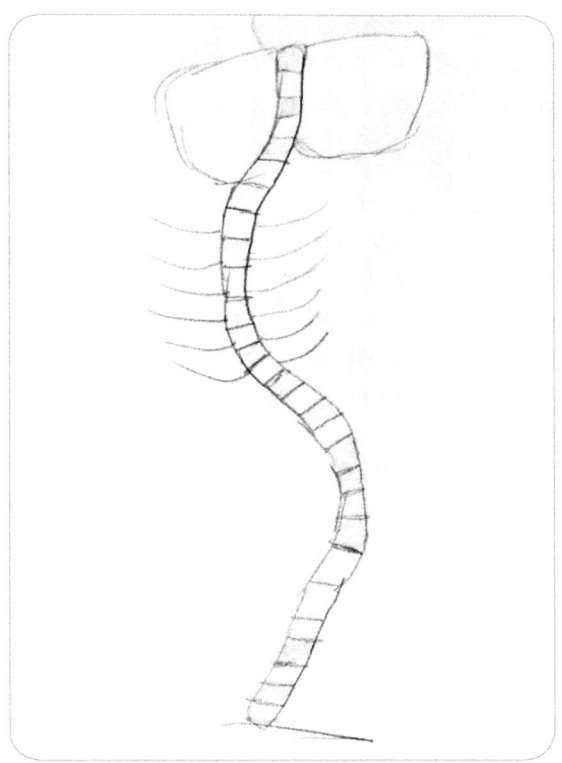

This case was surprising as one year later, the boy showed a spontaneous remission of his scoliosis: his x-ray presented a straight column. Talking to his mother, she told me they had never done any other treatment, but that at the moment he felt better, she separated from her husband, now she had a new partner with whom her son also had a good relationship. It was interesting to learn this background information considering the bio-psycho-social framework to connect his biography and scoliosis, avoiding any causal relationship.

I have invited adult patients to creative writing sessions, but it was very different: their voices were more filtered; there was not as much creative exploration, they talked about the needs of the body, of their desire to dance, their need to be pampered and enjoy life in a less symbolic and more conscious way. Here there are two stories from adults:

**Kundalineing** is the story written by a 57-year-old psychotherapist with very slight scoliosis.

*Kundalineing asks me some for more space, more stretching, more space between one vertebra and another one. It asks me to dance and express itself. Kundalineing knows about more space and movement. Only that movement is possible. It knows that this undulating movement that snakes freely make is possible. It asks me for space and time to snake, roll and unroll, dance, turn and stretch.*

**Earthworm,** the story from a 38-year-old psychologist, who had undergone an operation, still with severe scoliosis:

*There was a small earthworm that had traveled a lot and made a long journey full of curves, nooks and hidden places. This worm was wiser than it thought, worked very hard every day, but it did not listen to what it really needed. Until one day it realized that it should listen to its needs. The earthworm became aware and began to listen and take care of itself.*

## Children to adults: rites of passage

Currently, the physiological change in the pubertal growth has accelerated its onset by at least two years, due to improved nutritional, medical and environmental changes[130]. If, physiologically, it is easy to determine the beginning and end of adolescence, sociologically there is no consensus. This uncertainty is reflected in a confusion about adolescent expectations and family function. Previously, society promoted the adolescent development and family reorganization. Nowadays, there is a lack of clarity in the familial relationship: in the face of the accelerated physical development of their adolescents, some families expect more autonomy, when it is still psychologically premature for the adolescents, while other families appear stuck in outdated and inefficient patterns of functioning. This last behavior leads to parents treating adolescents as big babies, while they demand to be treated as adults, causing a struggle for power.

In case of scoliosis, adolescents may be "forced to extend (their) period of dependence on parents and physicians for medical care."[131] Non-adherence to scoliosis treatment could be seen as risky behavior, as well as rebellion against dependence and to the treatment regimen.

In traditional cultures, society created rites of passage in coming-of-age ceremonies to recognize the transition from childhood to adulthood[132]. A rite of passage presented three clear steps: 1. The separation from everyday activities with a

---

130   Quinn WH, Newfield NA, Protinsky HO. Rites of passage in families with adolescents. Fam Process. 1985 Mar;24(1):101-11.
131   Eliason MJ, Richman LC. Psychological effects of idiopathic adolescent scoliosis. J Dev Behav Pediatr. 1984 Aug;5(4):169-72.
132   Markstrom CA. Initiation ceremonies and rites of passage in Brown B, Prinstein M editors. Encyclopedia of Adolescence. San Diego, CA; US: Elsevier Inc.; 2011. Volume 2; p 152-159.

geographical distance from the family or village; the separation increased insecurity and facilitated passage to the second phase; 2. The transition: the initiate was forced out of a secure identity and pushed to an uncertain and unknown status; this transitional state was intermediate, an in-between phase, a "no man's land". In this state, some specific ordeals or tests of manhood or womanhood were often required. For boys, they included an element of danger, coping with a real risk; for girls, they could be related to a recognition of fertility and their capacity to give birth to a child; 3.The incorporation was a reassimilation of the individual into society with their newly acquired status and an ending ceremony where the community welcomed the adult into society.

Those rites of passages represented a change from which there was no turning back, an irreversible morphogenesis into a man or woman. They functioned as an end to their previous life, dying as a child in order to be born again as an adult, granting greater privileges, responsibility and power to adolescents. Rites of passage also rescued parents from operating as protectors of their children in eternity and assisted them in avoiding the compulsion of planning the adolescent's life. For children, they were a developmental opportunity to promote self-confidence and to achieve a sense of accomplishment.

Today, receiving house keys, qualifying for a driver's license, voting, etc. could be seen as the rites of passage society offers: they are symbols of the adolescent's arrival into adulthood. However, they are more private and inconsistent symbols, not related to a real new status of the adolescent, inhibiting family shifts.

Nevertheless, as the functions of those ceremonies were so powerful, Siegel, in his book *Brainstorming*, suggests that as adults we can collectively create rites of passage. Otherwise, with the disadvantages of the disappeared rites of passage, there is an increase in risky behaviors in adolescents as a substitute for the challenges of the transition phase.

So, why do we view the treatment of scoliosis as an obstacle of personal development in a maturational process for the adolescent patient? A physiotherapeutic treatment can be part of a transformational experience, combining physical exercises with the promotion of the patient's inner power, strength, self-knowledge and self-esteem. Being a Supportive Non-Parent Adult, a physical therapist is directly involved in this process, not only as an instructor but as an inspiring leader. A treatment based on exercises turns into an individual process for the patient, where the family participates in reinforcing the patient's, **only** in case of need. If the patients are adolescents who understand the treatment, they can learn exercises and be trained by the physiotherapists, without looking at their parent, otherwise they know that the parents will instruct them later and therefore they do not need to focus and learn the exercises themselves. That parental presence can keep the patient feeling like a helpless child who needs to be always supervised, continuing the dependence on the parents and stifling their self-confidence and autonomy.

## #5# Treatment as a rite of passage

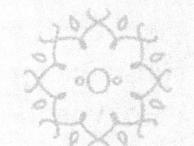

Rather than infantilizing the patient, the treatment can be a real process of independence and it could happen gradually, when you consider the patient mature.

As we said before, to be like a rite of passage, three steps are required:

1. Separation, spatially parents are invited to wait outside instead of being witness to their adolescent's movements. To engage parents' trust, strategies could be introduced, for example, showing parents the exercises for 10 minutes at the end of the session;
2. Transition: the ordeals are the exercises, proposed as advanced temporal challenges to train the patient's body and willpower;
3. Incorporation, at the end of treatment: a celebration with the whole family, friends and groups for the efforts accomplished and the results achieved.

For psychologists, I propose different work with adolescents, answering the question: *How do we become adults?*

## ♯6♯ From a Caterpillar to a Butterfly: a Vision Board

The work is aimed at the transition from childhood and the construction of a vision of the future.

To answer the question "How do adolescents imagine their future?", a journey to the past and coming back to the present can be of help.

The work consists of marking three different spaces in the room, representing their childhood, adolescence and adulthood. The patients go through the spaces as if they travel along a timeline, open to feelings, images, sounds, smells and objects related to the three periods. Food for thought are questions such as: *How are you travelling from childhood to adulthood? How does the body feel in this stage?*

Finally, the ritual consists of letting childhood go, getting rid of something that now is useless, and expressing a silent purpose related to becoming an adult, crossing a visible barrier. The rite of passage is performed in front of the group.

Later, everyone writes notes or draws their lived experience. Here is an example of the notes of an adolescent girl going through the three spaces, where photos, summer on the beach and a wedding dress represent respectively childhood, adolescence and adulthood.

...

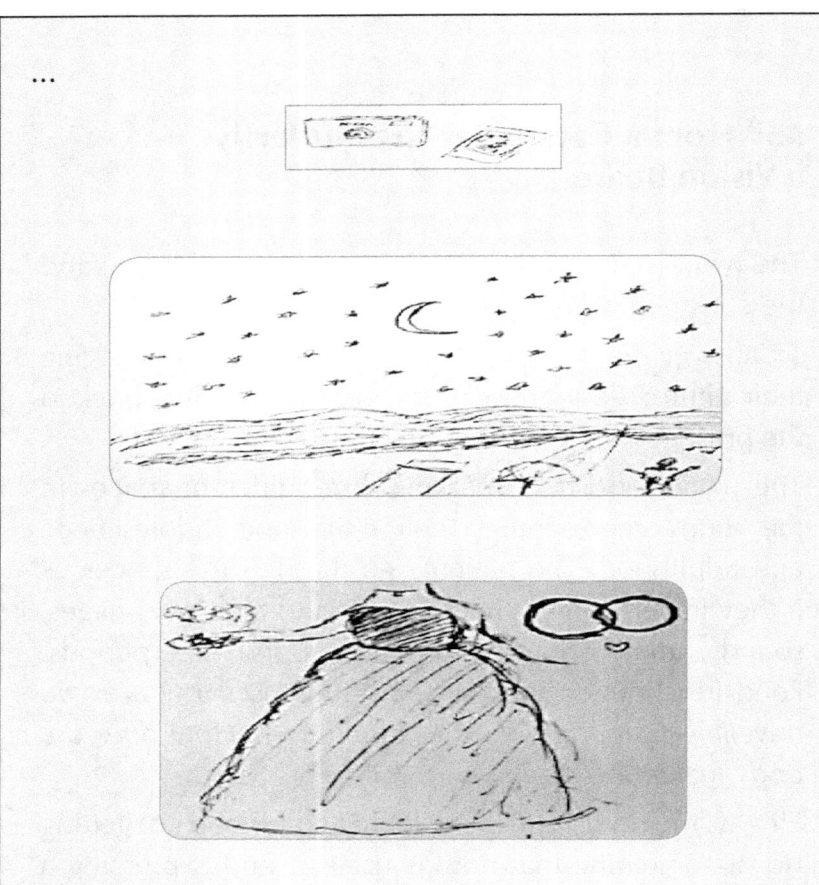

Every time this ritual is performed, it touches my heart: with bright eyes, an erect forehead and a heart full of desires, these teenagers move towards their future genuinely and seriously. It is a great honor to be a witness to this richness in their young age.

 In synthesis, the main points of this chapter are summarized below.

## The 10 Key Points of Chapter 5

1. Old and false myths have created a negative view of adolescence. They can have a limiting Pygmalion Effect on different areas of adolescent life, treatment included.
2. Thanks to recent neuroscience studies, we know that adolescence is a period that has the conditions to reach self-actualization. Four qualities describe the ESSENCE of adolescence: Emotional Spark, Social Engagement, Novelty Seeking and Creative Exploration.
3. Adolescents need the **presence** of adults. This presence is related to being receptive, open to what is happening, listening and tuning to the patient.
4. Adolescents create distance to separate themselves from their parents. Supportive Non-Parental Adults are important in the improvement of adolescents' self-esteem and conduct problems.
5. As professionals, our presence in their life could be of great importance to the adolescents.
6. As adults we need the presence of the adolescents to stay alive and in contact with the ESSENCE, avoiding falling into mundane routines, feeling alone and isolated, under the burden of the repetition.
7. Facebook pages used as discussion forums by patients with IS share pessimistic stories. Sad stories can limit the patient's power, while healthy stories are crucial to give life value.

8. Diseased stories can be replaced. The possibility of making one's own story is a central element of resilience. The story is about giving a shape to an image, repairing it. ♯1♯ *The story of the two Hunchbacks,* ♯2♯ *The poster,* ♯3♯ *A hunchback God* can be used as activities to reverse the trend, evoking empowerment and creativity, activating the ESSENCE of adolescence.
9. In traditional cultures, societies created rites of passage as coming-of-age ceremonies to recognize the transition from childhood to adulthood. Nowadays, these rites have disappeared, converted into inconsistent symbols to achieve a new identity for the adolescent.
10. Scoliosis treatment has been considered as a way to maintain dependence on parents. Rather than infantilizing the patient, the treatment could be a real part of the process of independence as in the activities ♯5♯ *Treatment as a rite of passage* or ♯6♯ *From the chrysalis to a butterfly.*

# Conclusion

*My secret is flying.*
*To fly you have to have wings,*
*like the ones my father built me.*
*They are wings made of flesh, feathers and wax;*
*heavy wings. (…)*
*I learned from seagulls and eagles,*
*they have big wings (...),*
*so they hover higher than everyone*
*and stare at the sun.*
**–D'Avenia**

## Inspiring our patients

It could be hard accompanying families and patients in this process of treatment full of insecurity and challenges. However, working with people with scoliosis could be extremely exciting if we try to listen to their voice and if they trust us to listen to them. While patients often complained of being uncomfortable, feeling different and unlucky compared to their friends, I would like to invite them to experience inner change, encouraging them to love themselves and their spine, despite its rotation. It would be beneficial to the adherence of treatment and to their self-esteem.

However, "How do you feel with your spine?" as well

as "How are you?" are not good questions: I realized the extremely discreet and shy nature of our spinal column, that only draws our attention in moments of pain, contractures, torsion and stiffness. So, I have thought about it over the years, attending workshops and also training myself and I have come to the conclusion that it is important to create a caring environment with specific activities to inspire our patients.

First of all, the setting is extremely important, as it communicates a certain quality of the treatment. The room where I worked in a hospital was the same one designated for occupational therapy, with a sink, a toilet and a bathtub. This environment did not help at all for that goal; the cold neon lights brought too much clarity to a situation that I wanted to approach in a different way. I desired to introduce an alternative to that "hygienic" environment. So, I sometimes turned on a softer light. I usually played classical music, often using music by Ludovico Einaudi or by Yan Tiersen to create a different environment. We often sat on the floor, as the chairs and the table seemed too static. The work changed in relation to the needs and aims of the patients, but it included body work, free movement, a circle of communication about ideas, feelings, etc.

Regarding activities, I used myths as means to help them construct positive images of themselves as travelers, explorers, creators and seekers of themselves, switching on their imagination, intuition, fantasy and artist side.

## The psychologist's role

*Should a braced teenager with scoliosis go to a psychologist?*

I have received this controversial question many times and there is no simple answer. Psychologists have two kinds of patients: people with psychopathological symptoms of suffering and people who are going through a difficult time. For the former, I hope no doubts exist when the adolescent is greatly suffering and presents clinical signs, such as anorexia, bulimia, self-harm, depression, insomnia, anxiety, claustrophobia, etc.

For all other cases, referring to those who are living in a stressful period in their life or those who would like to improve some aspects of their life, but do not have any associated psychopathology, it depends on a variety of factors. An essential element is the intrinsic motivation of the adolescents: the desire to change or to improve their life. If this is present, they are ready to start a process of change. In this case, the work is preventive, aimed at empowering the patients. People with scoliosis and a brace may belong to this second category, as they live a stressful life, they may need to reinforce their strategy of efficient coping mechanisms and resilience. In all of these cases, stress is not a disorder, rather it is a challenge that, if poorly handled, can lead to disorders. A brief and timely intervention can help people to deal with their situation.

For this reason, my aim has been to integrate a physiotherapist's role with the psychologist's role. A physiotherapist and a psychologist could work together, but in separate times, complementing one another's work with the patient, or a trained physiotherapist could learn tools to manage and transform stress, to connect with adolescent patients and their families, to reinforce adherence to the treatment and to create a channel of communication and trust.

This book is a work in progress; it does not give any definitive solution, only suggestions, food for thought, insights coming from my reflections and experience. Nowadays, we have the opportunity to apply a lot of knowledge from neuroscience, psychology, coaching and mindfulness techniques to the work of medical doctors, physiotherapists and orthopedic technicians, integrating compassion and science. Professionals should decide how extensively they want to do this integration in order to offer broader wellbeing to the patient. Independently of the techniques used, a warm connection is still the base of every treatment, as it is full of attention and of infinite possibilities, it may help our patients to feel free to flying according to their wishes and dreams.

The straight line belongs to men,
the curved one to God.

*Antoni Gaudi*

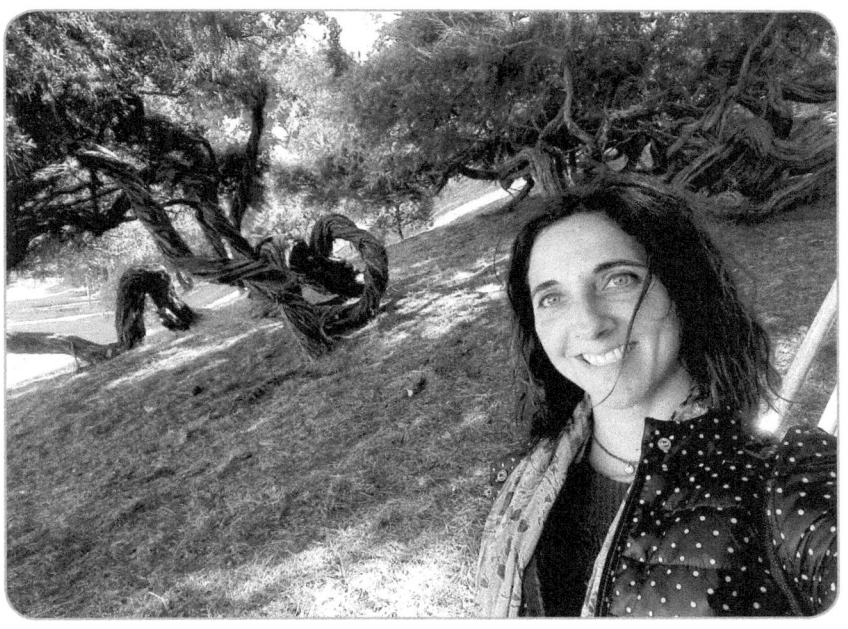

*From Golden Gate Park, San Francisco, CA*

www.ingramcontent.com/pod-product-compliance
Lightning Source LLC
Chambersburg PA
CBHW060852170526
45158CB00001B/324